The Cornea in Normal Condition and in Groenouw's Macular Dystrophy

The Cornea in Normal Condition and in Groenouw's Macular Dystrophy

Jules François
& Virgilio Victoria-Troncoso

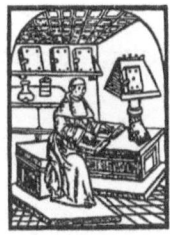

Dr. W. Junk bv Publishers The Hague-Boston-London 1980

Ophthalmological Clinic of the University of Ghent, Belgium.
Director: Professor Jules François.

Also published as volume 47 issue 2 of Documenta Ophthalmologica and supplied to its subscribers as part of their subscription.

ISBN-13: 978-94-009-9179-8   e-ISBN-13: 978-94-009-9177-4
DOI: 10.1007/ 978-94-009-9177-4

CONTENTS

VIII

ACKNOWLEDGEMENT

We would like to thank very warmly Dr. Enrique Malbran, who gave us some corneas affected by macular dystrophy and the facilities of his foundation. We also would like to thank very sincerely Mrs. Antoinette Victoria-Ihler, who prepared the tissue cultures, Mr. André Uvijls, who made the drawings, Mrs. Agnes Van Gerven, who prepared the electron-microscopical sections, and Mrs. Fanny Dhaenens, who typed the manuscript.

INTRODUCTION

The three most striking characteristics of the cornea are:

a) Its structure or rather its perfectly regular architectonic, by virtue of which it is transparent.

b) The absence of vessels, the cornea being nourished by the perilimbic vessels, the endothelial surface in communication with the aqueous humour and the epithelial surface in contact with the pre-corneal film.

c) The very slow turnover of the cells, that is to say the keratocytes, with the result that the metabolism of the cornea is very weak.

It is this third characteristic which justifies our present investigation.

The keratocytes, which are apparently inactive, have in fact a latent activity. They can be activated by central corneal incisions and also by tissue cultures. Under either of those conditions, the keratocytes become very active, develop all the cytoplasmic organites and produce mucopolysaccharides as well as the precursors of the collagen (Fig. 1).

In order to study the pathological keratocyte, we chose a storage disease, wherein the catabolism of the mucopolysaccharides is blocked, namely the macular dystrophy of the cornea.

We undertook the same investigation both for normal and for pathological corneas and studied the keratocyte 'in situ' and in tissue cultures using various microscopical and histochemical techniques. In macular dystrophy, we investigated also the deteriorations secondary to the changes in the keratocytes.

In view of the fact that, in macular dystrophy, the abnormality occurs at the level of the lysosomes, we undertook a comparative study 'in vitro' of the lysosomes of the keratocytes in tissue culture, obtained from normal corneas and from corneas affected by the disease.

Finally, we will discuss the pathogenesis and the treatment of macular dystrophy of the cornea.

We have not investigated the role of the keratocytes in inflammatory conditions of the cornea, which have already been fully developed by numerous authors.

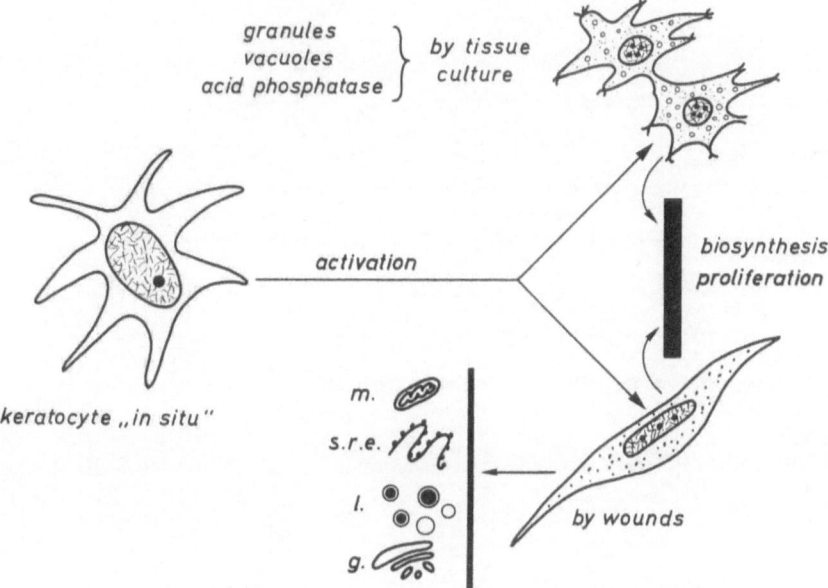

Fig. 1. Activation of the keratocyte by corneal wound or by tissue culture.

PART ONE

NORMAL KERATOCYTES

CHAPTER I

MATERIAL AND METHODS

Our investigation comprises five groups of histochemical and microscopical observations:

1) The study of the keratocyte *'in situ'.*
2) The study of the keratocyte behaviour in corneal wounds.
3) The study of the normal keratocyte in tissue culture.
4) The study of specimens of macular dystrophy of the cornea.
5) The study of macular dystrophy in tissue culture.

I. MATERIAL

For the study of the *keratocytes in situ*, we used 80 normal human corneas, as well as 183 corneas from adult, albinotic or pigmented rabbits (giants of Flanders). It must be borne in mind that the very young rabbits still have active keratocytes, which was not suitable for our investigations, which consisted in activating the keratocytes by a number of different methods.

For the study of the cicatrisation of the *corneal wounds*, we made, by means of a razor blade, a central corneal incision of from 3 to 4 mm, including the anterior half of the stroma.

The rabbits were dealt with under strictly sterile conditions; we washed their heads with a solution of lauryl sulphate, triethanolamine and chloro-5-hydroxy-2-diphenylmethane and instilled an antiseptic collyrium (non-antibiotic) in their eyes three times daily.

The experimental theatre was sterilised with UV light for twenty-four hours. We never operated upon more than three rabbits at one session. The animals were kept in the same theatre for forty-eight hours, in order to avoid infections.

As general anaesthetic, we used a mixture of fluanisone and phentanyl-citrate sub-cutaneously, in a dosage of 0.1 ml per 100 g of weight. It was necessary to wait fifteen minutes before obtaining complete narcosis. During that interval, the rabbit was hyperoxygenated with 98% oxygen.

We killed the rabbits by an injection of air in the marginal vein of the ear after the following delays: 0, 3, 6, 9, 12, 15, 18, 21, 24, 48 and 72 hours, 4, 8, 11 and 15 days, and 1, 2 and 3 months.

Each experiment comprised at least two rabbits. Only the right eye was incised, the left eye serving as control.

After the death of the rabbit, the ocular globe was enucleated and the cornea divided, as indicated in Fig. 2. Each piece was treated by the methods which will be described here below.

We placed the corneas of more than a hundred rabbits and of ten freshly removed human eyes *in culture*. The microscopical and histochemical study of the keratocyte culture, as well as their growth study, gave identical results in both cases.

We were able to examine ten corneas affected by macular dystrophy of the cornea, although this affection is very rare.

All these corneas were investigated histochemically and at the electron microscope. In three cases, we cultivated fragments of stroma, epithelium and endothelium.

II. METHODS

A. Histological and histochemical techniques

All the histological material, comprising the normal and pathological corneas and the implantation specimens, were treated in the same way.

1) *Fixation*. — We used the following fixatives:
a) 10% formol buffered with 0.06 M phosphate.
b) 10% formol buffered with phosphate, to which cetylpyridinium chloride was added, so that it had a final concentration of 0.5%. Cetylpyridi-

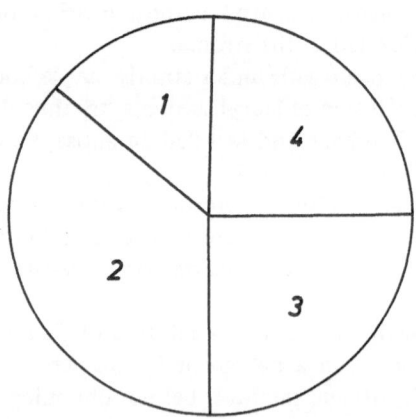

Fig. 2. Corneal segments intended for various microscopical studies:
1. Frozen sections; 2. Histopathology and histochemistry; 3. Transmission electron microscopy; 4. Scanning electron microscopy. Another fragment might be intended for tissue culture.

8

nium chloride is a quaternary ammonium salt, which precipitates the soluble mucopolysaccharides and makes thus their staining possible.

The average fixation time was twenty-four hours at 4°C.

2) *Dehydration*. — The specimens were immersed for two to three hours on an average, and even for as long as twelve hours for the bigger pieces, in the following baths:
   a) 50°, 60°, 70°, 80°, 90° and 96° alcohol, and thereafter
   b) absolute alcohol (three baths for at least three hours each),
   c) toluene (three baths for at least three hours each).

3) *Inclusion and sectioning*. — We used three baths of paraplast at 60°C for six hours each. The cornea was first placed vertically and, after successively cutting a number of sections depending upon the size of the specimen, the paraplastics substance was remelted and the specimen laid flat, in order to obtain seriated flat sections of 6 μm by means of a Reichert microtome.

4) *The removal of the paraffin and the rehydration* of the sections were effected in the conventional way: the sections were first heated and then hydrated by passing them through the following baths: toluene-toluene, absolute alcohol-absolute alcohol, then successively 90°, 80°, 70°, 60° and 50° alcohol, and finally distilled water.

5) *Frozen sections*. — We used the 'Cryo-cut' of the American Optical Company. The corneas are attached to the specimen-holder by a drop of glycerised water. According to our experience, the ideal temperature for corneal sections of 8 μm is − 28°C.

B. Culture techniques for normal keratocytes

We have developed our own technique for the keratocyte culture.

For the culture of the rabbit corneas, our procedure was as follows:
Preparation and culture of the corneal tissue

1) The rabbits were killed by an injection of 20 ml of air into the marginal vein of the ear.

2) The eyes were removed under sterile conditions and immediately washed twice with abundant physiological saline, for thirty minutes on each occasion.

The eyes were next immersed for an hour in a solution of penicillin (1 000 000 IU to 100 ml of physiological saline). This precaution was adequate, since we had no infection of the cultures.

3) The dissection of the eyes was carried out in a culture chamber sterilised by UV lamps, the usual surgical precautions being taken (disinfection of the hands, sterilised gloves and clothing, etc.).

The corneal epithelium was scratched with a knife, as in the peeling-off preliminary to keratoplasty. This operation has to be carried out carefully and slowly, in order to avoid contamination of the keratocyte cultures by the epithelial cells. After that, a very thin square strip of the stroma, measuring 2mm, was cut from the very centre of the cornea. This strip has to be as thin as possible, but it must not be torn. Those eyes which were accidentally perforated were eliminated, in order to avoid contamination by the anterior chamber cells.

We chose the central and anterior parts of the cornea, in order to have only keratocytes, and to avoid contamination by fibroblasts of other origins (conjunctiva or sclera).

The remainder of the ocular globe was dissected in order to obtain the hyalocytes, which were examined by the technique of François et al. (1972d) for the purpose of comparison of the cells.

4) The fragment of corneal stroma so obtained was placed against the wall of a T-flask or Leighton tube containing chicken plasma. The technique adopted is in fact the 'plasma-clot' technique. It is important that the surface of the implanted fragment shall not display any folds or curling of its edges. In some cases, the original square fragment was cut into smaller pieces, which were implanted in the same flask, but at places separated one from another.

The culture medium had the following composition:

Solution A:

TC medium 199 (Difco)	40%
Hanks B.S.S. solution (Difco)	40%
Chicken-embryo extract EE100 (Difco)	7.5%
Homologous serum	12.5%

The pH value was between 7.2 and 7.4

In order to improve the cultures, we added to the medium the precursors of the mucopolysaccharides and collagen.

Solution B:

L-proline	4.8 mg %
L-Hydroxyproline	1.2 mg %
Glycin	6 mg %
Glucose	2.5 mg %

Physiological saline up to 100 ml

To the culture flasks, the following medium was added:
a) For the Leighton tubes: 1 ml of solution A plus 0.1 ml of solution B.
b) For the T-flasks: 1.5 ml of solution A plus 0.15 ml of solution B.

The cultures were incubated at 37°C and inspected under the microscope at intervals of twenty-four hours.

10

Should the medium become too acid or too alkaline, it was changed immediately; normally it was changed twice weekly.

If the cells had grown sufficiently, a trypsinisation was effected on the sixth or the eighth day, and sub-cultures were made.

The trypsinisation was carried out in the following manner: (1) trypsinisation (0,2% trypsin 'Difco'), (2) centrifugation at 800 RPM. The supernatant was skimmed off and diluted in fresh medium.

This operation might be repeated.

The cells were re-implanted in suspension in the Leighton tubes or in the T-flasks, in order to obtain monolayers.

We did not make several successive sub-cultures to avoid cellular dedifferentiation.

Fixation of the cultures

Two fixatives were used:

a) 10% formol buffered with 0.06 M phosphate,

b) 10% formol buffered with phosphate, to which cetylpyridinium chloride was added in order to obtain a concentration of 0.5% of the latter in the buffered formol (formol-CPC).

These fixatives were added to the T-flasks after they had been washed with the 0.06 M phosphate buffer, or with the fixative itself. The fixation continued for from five to twenty-four hours.

One series of fresh monolayers was not fixed, but was mounted on a specimen-holder with a drop of Ringer's solution, before being examined.

Culture of human corneas

The normal and pathological human corneas were treated in the same way. First, we dissected, under sterile conditions, the anterior and posterior membranes, under the surgical microscope. Next, we cultivated separately the central and peripheral parts of the stroma, in view of the fact that the central part of the cornea contains almost exclusively keratocytes.

C. Technique for the study of the corneal architectonic

We used ten human eyes, around which we tightened threads, in such a way as to produce an increase in the ocular pressure and to maintain the cornea under pressure during the fixation, which was effected by means of neutral formol for at least twenty-four hours, the globes being dehydrated by alcohols of progressive concentration and xylol.

After the cornea had been removed, it was divided into small squares of 1 mm², as indicated in Fig. 3. Thus we obtained a central square, two paracentral squares and a paralimbic peripheral square. These pieces were enclosed in 'paraplast' by pressing them against the bottom of the recipient, so as to flatten them.

We made seriated flat sections, and three sections orientated in identical way were mounted on each specimen-holder. The paraffin was removed by two baths of xylol, and then covered with synthetic balsam (DPX).

The sections were examined at the (Wild) phase-contrast microscope and the (Zeiss) polarisation microscope. Measurements of the birefringence were made with the aid of $\lambda/4$ and $\lambda/2$ compensators. The microscopic methods are explained hereafter.

The centre of the first section was photographed, using the x20 objective, on to 36 mm negative film. A photograph of each of the other sections was taken at the same place. From each negative a 120 x 90 mm positive print was made.

On each of these prints, a line was drawn to indicate the orientation of the collagen bundles, and the angle formed by the bundles at one and the same level was measured, the variation of those angles being observed on different photographs. On the basis of the photographic analysis, a model could thus be devised.

Seriated transverse sections were examined in the same way in order to study the superposition of the lamellae and the structure of the corneoscleral zone at the limbus.

D. Histochemical techniques

a) *Routine histological techniques*
1) *Haematoxylin-eosin-saffron.* — We used Harris' haematoxylin-eosin in 1% aqueous solution and an alcohol solution of saffron prepared by distillation.
2) *Masson's and Gomori's trichromes.* — We used the methods recommended by the (U.S.A.) Armed Forces Institute of Pathology.

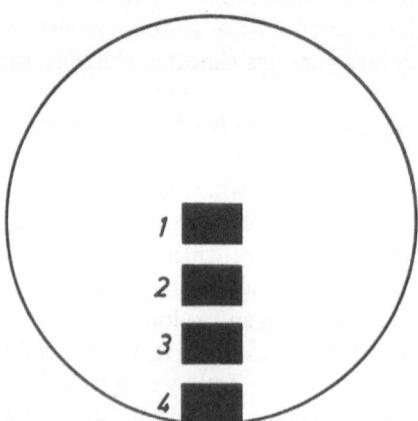

Fig. 3. Topographical study of the cornea with the aid of flat mountings: 1. Central, 2. and 3. paracentral, 4. peripheral.

12

b) *Staining of the collagen and its precursors*

1) *Van Gieson's method* (1% solution of acid fuchsin in a saturated solution of picric acid). – We have frequently used it without staining the nuclei, in order to observe the state of the collagen without artifacts.

2) *Reticulin.* – We used Wilder's method, as recommended by the Armed Forces Institute of Pathology.

c) *Staining for the mucopolysaccharides*

1) *Colloidal-iron method according to Rinehart and Abul-Haj (1951).* – The colloidal iron is fixed at the polyanionic surface of the mucopolysaccharides and the iron is identified by Prussian blue. We adopted the author's method without change.

2) *Alcian blue.* – We used this dye with various pH values:

a) 1% solution in 0.1N hydrochloric acid (pH 1). This solution gives a positive staining for the more sulphated mucopolysaccharides.

b) 1% solution in 3% acetic acid (pH 2.5). This solution gives a positive staining for sulphated and unsulphated mucopolysaccharides.

c) In some cases, we used diluted Alcian blue, buffered with phosphate and with pH values ranging from 1 to 8.

3) *Alcian blue and critical saline concentration.* – Magnesium chloride blocks the acid groups of the mucopolysaccharides, with the result that, the greater the number of free acid groups, the greater must be the saline concentration necessary to neutralise them and to prevent their staining by the Alcian blue.

We treated hydrated sections with increasing concentrations of magnesium chloride: 0.2M, 0.4M, 0.6M, 0.7M, 0.8M, 0.9M, 1.0M, 1.1M, 1.2M, 1.3M, 1.4M, 1.6M, 1.8M and 2.0M.

A set of serial sections was chosen for staining with pH 1 Alcian blue.

4) *Metachromatic curves according to François and Rabaey (1952).* – When a solution of toluidine blue or methylene blue is applied to a molecular surface more or less charged with anions, and when those anions are distributed periodically, the following results may be observed:

a) There are no anions, either they display no order or they are neutralised by a cation. In that case, the auxochrome groups of the dye adopt a random distribution and the resulting staining is orthochromatic, that is to say, that it displays the same blue colour as the dye.

b) There are many free acid groups, arranged periodically at 5Å intervals. This is, for example, the case of the highly sulphated mucopolysaccharides. In this case, a red-pink metachromasia is obtained, because there is a maximum of dye molecules. the auxochrome groups of which have a tendency to polymerise. There are three types of metachromasia: γ-metachromasia, which is the weakest, is purplish-blue; β-metachromasia is pink, and γ-metachromasia, which is the strongest, is pinker. Furthermore, by varying the pH value of the toluidine blue solution, the absorption of the dye by the polyanion can be determined (Fig. 4).

We slightly modified the technique of François et al., (1952):

(i) A series of eight hydrated sections was immersed in a solution of toluidine blue, each section having a different pH value. A 0.2M phosphate buffer was prepared, its monobasic phosphate and its dibasic phosphate being mixed, so as to obtain eight values of pH between 3 and 7.95. Of each such mixture, 9 ml were taken and mixed with 1 ml of a 0.5% aqueous solution of toluidine blue. Next, the eight sections were stained for three minutes with the toluidine blue solutions of increasing pH values.

(ii) Each section was then rinsed with the buffer of the same pH value.

(iii) The sections were mounted with a drop of the same buffer and a

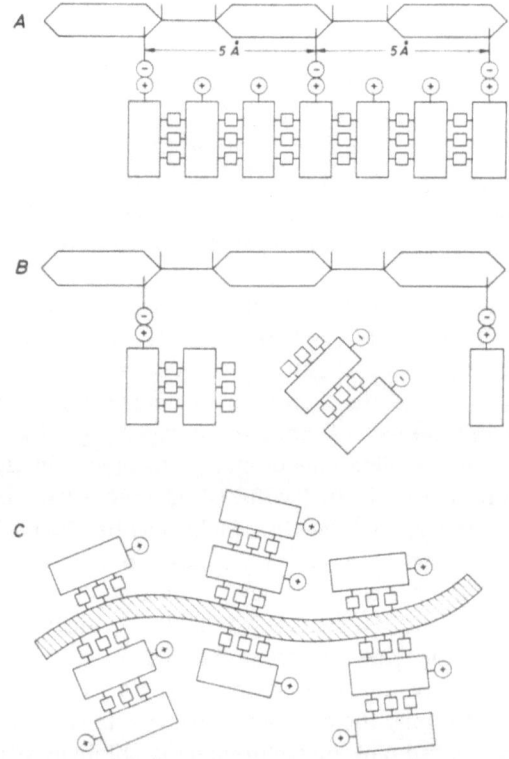

Fig. 4. Types of metachromasia: A. Along a mucopolysaccharide chain the groups are periodically arranged (periodicity of 5 Å in this example). The result is a regular arrangement of the molecules of the dye, which is polymerised, and a strong metachromasia (type β or γ); B. The acid groups are remote and few molecules can be orientated. The metachromasia is very weak (α-metachromasia). C. There are no acid groups, and the molecules of the dye are not orientated. The result is orthochromasia.

colour microphotograph was immediately taken under normal illumination (x 20 objective). The colour of the photographs was then analysed.

5) *Staining by acridine orange according to the method of Saunders (1964)*. — We adopted the method as recommended by the author. This technique is very specific for the determination of the types of mucopolysaccharides. The principle of the technique is set out in Chapter VII.

6) *Periodic-acid Schiff (PAS)*. — First, we tried the Schiff reagent without prior oxidation (direct Schiff). In every case, we used at least two different times of oxidation by the periodic acid — five and fifteen minutes — because in that way, the method becomes more sensitive. The acid mucopolysaccharides have, indeed, more accessible aldehyde groups, with the result that a shorter period of oxidation is necessary to make them evident.

We did not use dyes for the nuclei, because they very often mask weak positive results. We preferred to make direct observations under normal lighting or by phase contrast.

7) A 1% *Nile blue* aqueous solution has a certain affinity for the mucopolysaccharides, which are stained blue.

8) *Toluidine blue* in a 1% aqueous solution of aluminium sulphate produces a very intense metachromasia in the presence of mucopolysaccharides.

d) *Staining for lipids*

We used the classical techniques: Sudan III, Sudan black and Oil Red 'O'. For the cholesterol, we used the Schultze's reaction.

e) *Staining for the nucleic acids*

1) *Pyronine*. — Pyronine is specific for RNA only when a control is made with ribonuclease. We used a 0.5% aqueous solution.

2) *Method of Mortelmans and Sebruyns (1962)*. — We followed the authors' technique. With this method, the RNA takes on a red fluorescence and the DNA a green fluorescence.

f) *Staining for amyloid.*

We adopted the classical methods: Thioflavine 'T', Congo red and crystal violet.

g) *Histo-enzymological study*

Hyaluronidase test. — We used bovine testicular hyaluronidase ('Evans Rondase'), the concentration of which is 1 mg/ml in a 0.85% sodium-chloride solution. We treated one section with the solution containing hyaluronidase and another, serving as control, with the pure solvent. The two sections were then stained either with pH 6 toluidine blue or with pH 2.5 Alcian blue.

When hyaluronic acid or A or C chondroitin sulphate is present, the section treated with the hyaluronidase becomes negative for those stains, whereas the control section remains positive.

h) *Staining for acid phosphatase*

The phosphatases are enzymes which are very wide-spread in the organism. They act on the phosphate esters. The *acid phosphatases* are active at lower pH (less then 5) than the alkaline phosphatases. They have as substrate β-glycerophosphate, whereas the alkaline phosphatases have as substrate α-glycerophosphate. They are stored exclusively in the lysosomes, of which they constitute real markers.

1) *Takeuchi and Tanoue's method* for the acid phosphatases (Pearse, 1972), which is a modification of Gomori's classical method.

The substrate is β-glycerophosphate, which was prepared as follows:

2% sodium-β-glycerophosphate	2 vol.
0.1M acetate buffer (pH 5)	1 vol.
2% lead acetate	1 vol.
3% magnesium chloride	0.3 vol.

The monolayer was incubated in this solution for forty-five minutes at 37°C. It was then very quickly rinsed with distilled water and the cells immersed in ammoniacal silver nitrate for five to fifteen minutes, under microscopical control. As soon as the reaction became positive (dark brown to black staining), the photographs were taken. To avoid any precipitation, it was indispensable to use the incubation chamber that we described (François et al., 1972d).

2) *Standard azo-dye coupling method* for the acid phosphatases (Pearse, 1972). The substrate is sodium-α-naphthylphosphate. In 20 ml of 0.1M veronal acetate buffer (pH 5), 15 mg of the substrate was dissolved. Next, 1.5 mg of polyvinyl-pyrolidone were added and allowed to dissolve. Finally, 20 mg of Fast Red (ITR) were added and the solution filtered. The optimum incubation time was fifteen minutes at 37°C.

After rinsing, the cells were examined under the microscope, and microphotographs were taken. The positive staining was reddish brown. We did not stain the nuclei, which are, in any case, easily recognisable in the monolayer. Haematoxylin, indeed, masks the results.

(i) *Staining for β-glucuronidase*

We looked for the β-glucuronidase in the keratocytes activated by a corneal wound, as well as in the normal and pathological keratocyte cultures.

Staining technique. – We used the naphthol AS-BI glucuronide method described by Pearse (1972), which we slightly modified. We proceeded as follows. Frozen sections or monolayers were incubated for ten to fifteen minutes in the following solution:

Solution A: 28 mg of naphthol AS-BI glucuronide were dissolved in 1.2 ml of a 50 nM solution of sodium bicarbonate (420 mg of sodium bicarbonate in 100 ml of distilled water).

To this solution was added a 0.2N acetate buffer (pH 5), to make the volume up to 100 ml.

Solution B:

Pararosanilin hydrochloride	1 g
Distilled water	20 ml
Concentrated hydrochloric acid	5 ml

This solution was heated, filtered and then recooled.

Solution C: This is a 4% solution of sodium nitrite in distilled water.

Solution D: First, 0.3 ml of solution B was mixed with 0.3 ml of solution C. After one minute, 10 ml of solution A were added. By adding a normal solution of sodium hydroxide, the pH value was adjusted to 5.2. Finally, distilled water was added to make the volume up to 20 ml.

Result: A reddish colour is obtained when the pararosanilin associated with the substrate is bound at the places where there is a β-glucuronide activity.

j) *Staining for the α- and β-galactosidases*

The substrate for the β-galactosidase was prepared as follows: 100 mg of 6-bromo-2-naphthyl-β-D-galactopyranoside were dissolved in the following solution:

Methanol	15 ml
Phosphate-citrate buffer (pH 4.95)	85 ml

The 4.95 pH phosphate-citrate buffer was obtained by mixing 0.2 M disodium phosphate (1 part) with 0.1 M citric acid (1 part). Lastly, distilled water was added to make the volume up to 100 ml.

The frozen sections and the monolayers were incubated at 37°C in this solution for between forty-five minutes and one hour. Next, they were rinsed with distilled water and stained for ninety seconds with an aqueous solution of Fast Blue (concentration 1 mg/ml) at 4°C and pH 7.4. Finally, they were rinsed with distilled water at 4°C.

Result: The positive places take on a blue staining, because the enzyme/substrate complex specifically takes this dye.

The method for the α-galactosidase is similar, but in that case, the substrate is 6-bromo-2-naphthyl-α-D-galactopyranoside.

k) *Standard method for the glucose-6-phosphate dehydrogenase*

First, three solutions have to be prepared:

Solution A (stock solution):

Aqueous solution of nitro BT (4 mg/ml)	2.5 ml
Tris-buffer (pH 7.4)	2.5 ml
5nM solution of magnesium chloride	1 ml
Distilled water	3 ml

Solution B (substrate stock solution):

Disodium-glucose-6-phosphate	3.04 g
Distilled water	8 ml
Normal solution of hydrochloric acid	0.6 ml
Distilled water	to 10 ml

Solution C:

Solution A	0.9 ml
Solution B	0.1 ml
100 nM sodium chloride	0.1 ml
Polyvinylpyrolidine	75 mg
Phenasine methosulphate	1mg/ml of solution
DNA	2mg/ml of solution

The frozen sections or the monolayers were incubated in the dark at 37°C for fifteen minutes in solution C. If, after a microscopical examination, it was found that the staining was insufficient, the incubation could be continued for up to forty minutes. Finally, the specimens were rinsed, first with tap water and afterwards with distilled water.

Result: The stained substrate is bound at the places of enzymatic activity and gives them a dark-blue coloration.

1) *Lactic dehydrogenase*

We used Hanker's osmium-tetroxide method, as described by Pearse (1972). The substrate was prepared as follows:

0.5M potassium tartrate	6 ml
0.1M phosphate buffer (pH 7.4)	1.6 ml

After mixing for several minutes, the following was added:

0.3M copper sulphate	0.7 ml
10M lactic acid	0.025 ml
DNA	5 mg
Dimethyl sulphoxide	1.5 ml

The pH value was adjusted to between 6.6 and 6.8. Before using 0.3 ml of 2% potassium ferrocyanide was added drop by drop. The incubation was effected at 37°C for between thirty and thirty-five minutes.

Next, the substrate was rinsed with 40% formaldehyde in a 0.1 M phosphate buffer and fixed in that solution for two hours.

After fixing, the material was treated for several minutes with 0.5% thiocarbohydrazide. Finally, after rinsing with distilled water, the osmium tetroxide (2% aqueous solution) was applied at 50°C for five minutes.

Result: The osmium tetroxide is bound to the substrate by osmium bridges and stains the places of enzymatic activity brown.

m) Experience concerning the presence of a catabolic substance in the homogenates of normal keratocytes and capable of acting on the mucopolysaccharides stored in macular corneal dystrophy, is set out in Chapter XV.

n) *Method for studying lysosomes 'in vitro' after vital staining with acridine orange*

We were the first to apply this method to ocular tissue cultures. We modified the technique of Allison et al. (1973).

Staining technique. — The primary cultures and subcultures of normal and pathological keratocytes were treated as follows:

(1) Incubation of the cells in a medium containing a concentration of $1:10^5$ (P/V) of acridine orange per millilitre of the culture medium. The optimum time of staining was eight minutes.

(2) Rinsing for from two to three minutes with a medium containing no dye.

(3) Mounting of the monolayer on a specimen-holder with the aid of a drop of the culture medium.

(4) If the staining was insufficient, the monolayer might be put back in a Leighton tube and the staining repeated for two or three minutes. After that, (2) and (3) were repeated.

III. DISCUSSION

We should like to discuss, on the one hand, the microscopical and histochemical methods of detecting two essential macromolecules of the corneal stroma, which are synthesised by the keratocytes: namely, the acid mucopolysaccharides and the collagen. We should like also to discuss, on the other hand, the methods for detecting two organelles which are relevant to our study: namely, the lysosomes and the mitochondria. In the second case, we used methods for localising the particles, as well as methods for demonstrating those enzymes that are most relevant to our study.

A) Mucopolysaccharides

To demonstrate the mucopolysaccharides, we have used numerous histochemical methods, as well as topo-optical methods, which make possible an analysis of their macromolecular structure. Methods based on PAS, Alcian blue or colloidal iron have long been described. However, it has been only during the last five years, that they have acquired a greater precision, thanks to a better knowledge of their action mechanism.

1) *Biochemical bases*

Some of the physico-chemical properties of the mucopolysaccharides constitute the basis of the histochemical reactions, both under the optical microscope and under the electron microscope.

The most important are the following:

a) It is always necessary to bear in mind the fact that the mucopolysaccharide chains behave exactly as macromolecules. All their biological properties are based on this 'structured' behaviour.

The mucopolysaccharides behave, indeed, like long chains of macromolecules, which are capable of linking with either collagen or non-collagenous proteins, to form structured elements.

b) The acid groups of the mucopolysaccharides are more or less ionised, that is to say, that they have free negative charges.

$$CO.OH \;\text{———————————}\; CO.O^- + H^+$$
$$SO_3H \;\text{———————————}\; SO_3^- + H^+$$

When the long polysaccharide chain is considered, it is readily understood that the free acid groups are very numerous; in other words, it is a matter of polyanions. When there is an association of polyanionic chains, it may be described as a *polyanionic surface* (Figs. 5 and 6).

The degree of ionisation depends upon the pH value of the medium; it decreases with decreasing pH values. This property is of capital importance, because it is fundamental for certain methods of chemical and histochemical investigation. Furthermore, the normality of the corneal structure depends to a large extent upon the integrity of that equilibrium, the breakdown of which gives rise to pathological phenomena, for example, in congenital oedematous dystrophy of the cornea (Victoria-Troncoso et al., 1969).

c) The mucopolysaccharides have no reducing capability.

d) As a result of their polysaccharide character, the mucopolysaccharides are unable to produce colloidal solutions.

e) The length of the chains, as well as the more or less *periodic* distribution of the negative charges, play a capital role in the majority of the histochemical reactions.

f) The oxidation of the hexoses by, for example, periodic acid, breaks the links of each hexose molecule between C2 and C3; an aldehyde group is liberated for each of those carbon atoms.

g) The formation of chemical complexes with the quaternary ammonium salts. There is a critical point in the concentration of the quaternary ammonium salts, beyond which the salts no longer dissolve. If a polyanion, such as the mucopolysaccharides, is introduced into the solution, a certain

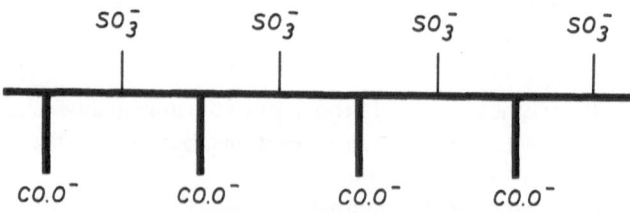

Fig. 5. Mucopolysaccharide chain, in which the negative charges of the sulphated and carboxyl groups repeat periodically.

quantity of the ammonium salts fixes on the negative charges. This quantity will be the greater, to the extent that the anionic surface contains more negative charges. At that moment, the *critical concentration* of the ammonium salts seems to increase. If this concentration is determined before and after the introduction of the mucopolysaccharides, the quantity of anions introduced into the solution can be measured.

The sulphated acid mucopolysaccharides will produce a greater change in the critical concentration of the ammonium salts than do the non-sulphated acid mucopolysaccharides, which, being less acid, constitute a weaker polyanion.

To sum up, this method determines the mucopolysaccharides according to their negative charges. The sulphated mucopolysaccharides give more

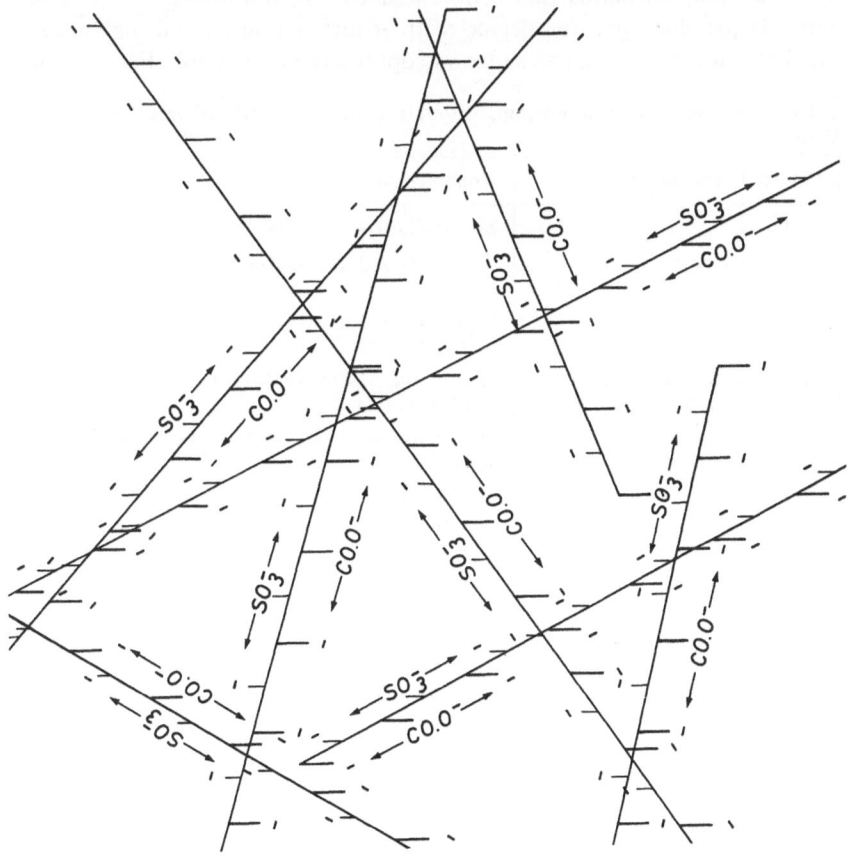

Fig. 6. Polyanionic 'surface' formed by the overlapping of several chains.

evident results, because they have a larger number of negative charges to act on the ammonium salts.

h) The *precipitation of the mucopolysaccharides* can be brought about by introducing them into a solution whose pH value permits the presence of a large number of positive charges capable of neutralising the anions of the polysaccharide chain. If the ionic strength necessary to neutralise the negative charges of the mucopolysaccharides under study is measured, similar results to those arrived at by the quaternary ammonium salt method can be obtained. A greater ionic strength (a more alkaline pH value) is necessary for neutralising the sulphated acid mucopolysaccharides than for neutralising the non-sulphated acid mucopolysaccharides.

i) As will be indicated below, the mucopolysaccharides display, under certain conditions, optical anisotropy.

2) *Biosynthesis of the mucopolysaccharides at the level of the cell*

The mucopolysaccharides are synthesised by the fibroblasts of the mesoderm. Depending upon the degree of their differentiation and their genetic message, they produce a particular mucopolysaccharide 'pool'. For example,

Table 1. Mucopolysaccharides composition (according to BRIMACOMBE and WEBBER, 1964).

Mucopolysaccharides	Monosaccharides
Chitin	2-acetamido-2-desoxy-D-glucose
Hyaluronic acid	(2-acetamido-2-desoxy-D-galactose) D-glucuronic acid
Chondroitin	(2-acetamido-2-desoxy-D-galactose) D-glucuronic acid
Chondroitin sulphate A (chondroitin-4-sulphate)	(2-acetamido-2-desoxy-4-*O*-sulpho-D-galactose) D-glucuronic acid
Chondroitin sulphate B (dermatan sulphate)	(2-acetamido-2-desoxy-4-*O*-sulpho-D-galactose) L-iduronic acid
Chondroitin sulphate C (chondroitin-6-sulphate)	(2-acetamido-2-desoxy-6-*O*-sulpho-D-galactose) D-glucuronic acid
Heparin	(2-desoxy-2-sulphoamino-D-glucose) D-glucuronic acid (both molecules are *O*-sulphated)
Keratosulphate (keratan sulphate)	(2-acetamido-2-desoxy-6-*O*-sulpho-D-glucose) D galactose
Heparitin sulphate (heparan sulphate)	(2-desoxy-2-sulphoamino-D-glucose (containing also *O*-sulphated groups) -2-acetamido-2-desoxy-D-glucose) D-glucuronic acid
Teichuronic acid (teichone)	(2-acetamido-2-desoxy-D-galactose) D-glucuronic acid
Blood groups substances	L-fucose, D-galactose, 2-acetamido-2-desoxy-D-glucose, 2-acetamido-2-desoxy-D-galactose

the keratocytes produce above all keratosulphate, the hyalocytes produce hyaluronic acid, and so on (Table I).

It is already certain that the mucopolysaccharides are synthesised in the Golgi's apparatus or dyctyosome of the cells. The Golgi's apparatus, as studied at the electron microscope, is seen to be composed of membranous elements: (1) flattened cisterns, arranged in such a fashion that together they present one concave and one convex face, and (2) small vesicles which merge to produce bigger vacuoles (Favard, 1969; Threadgold, 1969; Neutra et al., 1969; De Robertis et al., 1970).

The Golgi's apparatus has a lipoproteic chemical composition, intermediate between that of the reticulo-endoplasmic system and that of the cell membrane. That fact has been demonstrated, as isolated Golgi's apparatus have been obtained. Cationic colloidal thorium, which is a cytochemical dye for the polyanions (such as the mucopolysaccharides), is fixed in the larger vacuoles of the Golgi's apparatus (Revel, 1970). The cytochemical stainings, however, do not indicate that the Golgi's apparatus must be the place where the mucopolysaccharides are biosynthesised. It is known that some other chemical compounds, such as Trypan blue, also accumulate in the Golgi's apparatus, without, nevertheless, having any connection with the biosynthesis of the mucopolysaccharides. Certain more precise methods, such as the oxidation by chromic acid or a periodate (Rambourg et al., 1969), have demonstrated that a weaker positivity exists at the level of the Golgi's cisterns, the staining being more positive on the concave side than on the convex side. Revel (1970) concluded that only the 'mature' elements of the Golgi's apparatus are stained by the dyes that need to have a large polyanionic surface, such as those of the sulphated mucopolysaccharides (Fig. 6). The weaker cytochemical dyes indicate less polymerised and non-sulphated chains accumulated in the 'less mature' parts.

The autoradiographical methods show, nevertheless, not only that mucopolysaccharides may be found in the Golgi's apparatus, but also that this is the seat of their biosynthesis. These techniques utilise, on the one hand, the incorporation of S^{35} (Goldman et al., 1964; Revel, 1970) and of H^3-acetate (Revel, 1970) and, on the other hand, the incorporation of glucose and of galactose (Peterson et al., 1964; Neutra et al., 1966; Revel, 1970). At the electron microscope, it can be seen that the incorporation of radioactive substances occurs at the level of the Golgi's apparatus, and it can at the same time be demonstrated chemically that the radioactive substance is a mucopolysaccharide. Revel (1970) also observed that the synthesised material appeared *immediately* in the Golgi's apparatus. If the mucopolysaccharides, the precursors of which had been marked, were synthesised in the reticulo-endoplasmic system and then moved into the Golgi's apparatus, it would be only half an hour later that the latter would appear radioactive, as is the case, for example, for the synthesised proteins, studied by means of marked aminoacids.

23

All of the synthesised mucopolysaccharide material tends to reach the interstitial matrix. Studies on this subject have been made on cartilage cells.

The incorporation *'in vitro'* in the culture flask, has been studied for several types of fibroblasts.

It is believed, moreover, that the vacuoles are more active than the vesicles, and that the cisterns are less active.

De Robertis et al. (1970) thought that, in general, the carbohydrates are synthesised from monomers in the Golgi's apparatus, where their sulphation also occurs.

The new mucopolysaccharides can link up with the proteins synthesised by the ribosomal reticulo-endoplasmic system, to form glycoproteins.

Thanks to the study of isolated Golgi's apparatus, it has been possible also to observe that they contain enzymes capable of linking the mucopolysaccharides to the proteins (UDP-N-acetyl-glycosamine-transferase, galactosyl-transferase and others: De Robertis et al., 1970).

The problem of the biosynthesis of the mucopolysaccharides by the Golgi's apparatus was discussed by Neutra et al. (1969).

In conclusion, the morphological and cytodynamic study of the Golgi's apparatus can provide indirect information about the biosynthesis of the mucopolysaccharides; as we shall see later, the Golgi's apparatus was hypertrophied in the mucopolysaccharidosis that we have studied.

3) *Histochemical reactions for the study of the mucopolysaccharides*
There are many problems to be solved, in connection with the histochemical study of the mucopolysaccharides; they may be summarised as follows:

a) *Determination of the existence of a mucopolysaccharide.* In this case, methods are required that are sufficiently selective to be able to differentiate between the mucopolysaccharides and other substances also having hydrocarbon chains.

b) Determination whether a mucopolysaccharide is *sulphated*.

c) If it is sulphated, it is necessary to differentiate between the *different types*. In the case of the cornea, the most difficult problem is that of differentiating between chondroitin sulphate B and keratosulphate.

d) Finally, it is necessary to study the *macromolecular organisation* of the polysaccharide chains.

The literature on the histochemistry of the mucopolysaccharides is very extensive. It is for that reason that only recent work and methods concerning our investigation will be discussed here.

a) *Histochemical determination of the presence of a mucopolysaccharide.* — A mucopolysaccharide can exist in a soluble or in an insoluble state. Fixatives in aqueous solution eliminate the soluble mucopolysaccharides and thus prevent positive stainings; it is necessary in those circumstances to use appropriate fixatives. In the case of insoluble mucopolysaccharides,

24

although there will always be a certain amount of extraction, the usual fixatives give good results without prior treatment.

Elleder (1976) compared several methods of fixation, in order to retain the soluble hydrocarbonated chains of the mucopolysaccharides in the tissues. The author found that the best results were obtained by fixing in 99° methanol and staining with Azure A. Lojda (1974) obtained less satisfactory results when ethanol was used as fixative. We used fixatives containing cetylpyridinium chloride which, as we have already mentioned, precipitate 'in situ' the soluble mucopolysaccharides; this method has been used for the study of the soluble mucopolysaccharides of the cornea by Kitano (1966, 1969) and by Kitano et al. (1966).

For the fixation of the insoluble mucopolysaccharides, fixation with neutral formol or with glutaraldehyde is sufficient.

When, at the outset, it is not known which mucopolysaccharides will be encountered, it is preferable to use systematically cetylpyridinium chloride. It seems, however, that the tissues treated with cetylpyridinium chloride display weaker stainings (Elleder, 1976).

What techniques ought to be applied?

We made first of all a PAS , which enabled us to localise the places where there were hydrocarbonated chains. Such a study was indispensable before the application of topo-optical methods.

Puchtler et al. (1975) were able to establish the formula of Schiff's reagent; it is a tri-aminophenylmethane, whose resonance formula permits two or three free charges. Furthermore, oxidation by periodic acid gives the best results, when concentrations ranging from 0.01 to 0.005% are used, that is to say, distinctly less than those usually used, which are in the neighbourhood of 0.5 to 1% (Pearse, 1972).

Alcian blue belongs to the phythalocyanin group. It is more specific for the mucopolysaccharides (Pearse, 1972). It combines as readily with sulphated and non-sulphated polyanions as with the sulphatide groups (Lampert et al., 1975). The chemical mechanism was described by Scott (1973).

Colloidal iron fixes very strongly on polyanionic surfaces. The iron can be localised histochemically with the aid of Prussian blue or, thanks to its electron density, at the electron microscope; this method is very sensitive. In this manner, for example, Mareel et al. (1976) studied the polyanion of the cell membrane of the HeLa cells and the erythrocytes. The negative charges are provided either by an acid polysaccharide chain or by the sialic acids. It has to be recalled that the histochemical method has been described by Hale (1946) and applied at the electron microscope by Gasic et al. (1963).

The metachromasia with toluidine blue has already been discussed.
That method is comparable with the metachromasia obtained with Azure A, the mechanism of which is similar. The latter, however, stains the soluble mucopolysaccharides more satisfactorily (Elleder, 1976).

25

b) *Identification of the type of mucopolysaccharides.* – Several methods have been described as being more or less selective for one mucopolysaccharide or another. All the methods have one feature in common: they measure the polyanionic surface and detect the presence of sulphated groups. Moreover, enzymatic digestion makes it possible to eliminate certain mucopolysaccharides that are sensitive to it.

The use of pH 1 Alcian blue (Lev et al., 1964) and of pH 2.5 Alcian blue (Pearse, 1972) already renders possible a preliminary differentiation between, on the one hand, the sulphated mucopolysaccharides, which are well stained at pH 1 and weakly at pH 2.5, and, on the other hand, the non-sulphated mucopolysaccharides, as well as the sialomucins, which are stained at pH 2.5. Paradoxically, the most acid mucins stain more weakly at pH 1.

Alcian blue at pH 5.8 with increasing concentrations of magnesium chloride was used by Spicer et al. (1967). This method is based upon the blocking of the polyanionic surface by a critical saline concentration which inhibits the positivity of the staining. We have already discussed the mechanism of the critical saline concentration, as well as the results of the metachromatic curves, which are of great utility.

Other methods of blocking are saponification and methylation, which we have not used.

Some examples of the association of different techniques are to be found in the papers of Rovasio et al. (1974), Yamada et al. (1975) and Yamada et al. (1976).

Enzymatic digestion renders it possible to eliminate certain muco-substances: bacterial amylase (Yamada, 1965), neuraminidase (Spicer et al., 1967) and hyaluronidase (Pearse, 1972). The last-mentioned enzyme acts on the hyaluronic acid and on the chondroitin sulphates A and C.

c) The chondroitin sulphates A and C can be eliminated by digestion with hyaluronidase, but in order to differentiate the chondroitin sulphate B from the keratosulphate, a problem which concerns the cornea especially, we used the method of Saunders (1964), which gave us very satisfactory results. Recently, Sames (1974) introduced a method which associates Alcian blue and acridine orange; this method is combined with the determination of the critical saline concentration with the aid of magnesium chloride.

d) *Determination of the macromolecular structure of the mucopolysaccharides.* – Much information about the macromolecular structure of the mucopolysaccharides is obtainable by associating the stainings where the molecules of the dye are oriented in a particular fashion, and the polarisation microscopy, which enables to study the crystalline structures thereby formed. Such methods are termed topo-optical.

Two macromolecules can be studied by this method in the normal or pathological cornea: (1) the collagen, the characteristics of which we shall discuss later, and (2) the mucopolysaccharides and, indeed, any polysaccharide chain.

It is also possible to investigate the macromolecular structure of the cell membranes, as well as the structural glycoproteins which are found in the connective tissue. The cornea, which has a very specialised macromolecular organisation, lends itself most particularly to topo-optical research.

Topo-optical reactions for the study of histological material were introduced by Schmidt (1947).

Those methods were improved by the School of Pathological Anatomy at the University of Budapest (Romhányi, 1949 and 1963; Romhányi et al., 1969, 1973, 1974a, 1974b, 1974c and 1975). Other researchers have applied the method to the study of various biological tissues (Schmidt, 1947; Movat, 1961; Mowry, 1963; François et al., 1972a, 1972b and 1972c; Musy et al., 1972; Scheuner et al., 1972; Módis, 1974; Vidal et al., 1974).

What is the principle of the topo-optical methods as applied to the study of the mucopolysaccharide chains?

The current histochemical methods, such as PAS, or the electron microscope, make it possible to demonstrate the neighbouring hydroxyl groups, for example, those of C2 and C3 in the molecules of hexose. It is nevertheless necessary that these hexoses form part of a chain that has a certain macromolecular stability. The literature concerning the demonstration of the hydroxyl groups in the hydrocarbonated chains is very extensive and will not be discussed here. The histochemical methods do not, however, produce optical anisotropic phenomena, and as a consequence do not give any information about the macromolecular arrangement of the hydrocarbonated chains or about the structures to which those chains are attached. The topo-optical reactions do make it possible to solve that problem; the principle of the method is as follows (Romhányi et al., 1973; Romhányi et al., 1975):

a) The oxidation to dialdehydes of two neighbouring hydroxyl groups (for example, the C2 and C3 of a hexose) is effected by periodic acid.

b) By the addition of bisulphite, the dialdehydes are sulphated and as a consequence become charged negatively.

c) These sulphated hydrocarbonated chains can be stained by pH 1 toluidine blue. The result is, on the one hand, a basophilia and, on the other hand, an optical anisotropy, which can be measured at the polarisation microscope equipped with a compensator.

d) The structure is stabilised by potassium ferrocyanide. Romhányi (1963) demonstrated that it stabilises the metachromasia of the substances that display labile or unstable metachromasia.

If the substance displays already a large number of negative charges arranged periodically, as in the case of keratosulphate, that is to say, if

27

metachromasia is obtained at pH 1 without preliminary treatment, the procedure is then as follows:

(i) Reversal of the sign of the birefringence of the collagen by phenol reaction.

(ii) Study of the anisotropy of the naturally-sulphated mucopolysaccharide chains at the polarisation microscope equipped with a compensator.

Thanks to the topo-optical methods, it was possible to determine three types of structures.

1) *Arrangement of the hydrocarbonated chains in the cell membranes (Romhányi et al., 1974c).* − Certain membranes, such as those of the erythrocytes, display, after topo-optical staining with pH 6 toluidine blue, positive dichroism with a maximum of absorption in the direction of the ray which corresponds to positive radiary dichroism. That fact indicates that the molecules of toluidine blue are radiarily oriented relative to the surface of the membrane. In view of the fact that the molecules of toluidine blue are perpendicularly fixed to the hydrocarbonated chains, it may be deduced that the latter are arranged parallel to the membrane surface. Between the polariser and the analyser, the membrane display a strong continuous birefringence, positive relative to the cell surface and negative relative to the hydrocarbonated chains.

The arrangement of the isotropic phenomena by extraction of the lipids by methanol-chloroform indicates that the hydrocarbonated chains are attached to the lipid component of the membrane.

Another example is that of the lymphoid cells, which display an irregular birefringence, distributed in 'granules' along the membrane. That birefringence increases and becomes continuous after the addition of periodic acid bisulphite. This addition gives rise, on the contrary, to a diminution of the birefringence in the erythrocytes. That phenomenon is explained as follows (Romhányi et al., 1974c). In the case of the erythrocytes, the birefringence decreases as a result of the collapse of the delicate molecular structure of the glycoproteins at the level of the external hydrophilic zone of the membrane. The 'granular' appearance of the birefrigence is due to a derangement in the orientation of the dye molecules.

In the case of white globules, the augmentation of the birefringence after treatment with periodic acid bisulphite indicates an increase of the negative charges in the hydrocarbonated chains, arranged tangentially. It is possible that in this case the hydrocarbonated chains form part of the glycolipids, which do not have free negative charges.

2) *Long chains*, which are attached to the structural glycoproteins. These chains are found in large numbers in the corneal stroma at the level of the ground substance (François et al., 1972a, 1972b and 1972c; Romhányi et al., 1973). Two problems arise: (i) the strong birefringence of the adjacent collagen and (ii) the determination of the arrangement of the mucopo-

lysaccharide chains. In the first case, the sign of the birefringence of the collagen is reversed by the phenol reaction.

The arrangement of the chains is determined by the study of the birefringence of the polysaccharide chains linked with the molecules of toluidine blue, which, as we have pointed out, are perpendicularly and periodically arranged relative to the length of the chain.

3) When the polysaccharide chains are stored in the granules, a red polarisation colour is obtained, which indicates a certain disorder in the molecular structure. The birefringence is irregular, because the polysaccharide chains are of different lengths and are in many cases ramified. Furthermore, the chains are superposed one on another. The molecules of toluidine blue, which are perpendicularly arranged to each chain, are also obliged to superpose. The result is then a birefringence of negative sign, the image of which is far from distinct.

It may be concluded that the hydrocarbonated chains are arranged in the superposed fascicles within the granules, in such a fashion that together they constitute a paracrystalline structure (Romhányi et al., 1975). The granules of mucopolysaccharide thesaurismosis like those described in Chapter VI, constitute an example of the structure that we have just described.

B) Collagen and reticulin

The collagen consists of non-ramified fibres which are stained red by the Van Gieson method, pink by the PAS method, blue by the sulphation metachromasia method, brown by silver impregnation and yellow by saffron. At the polarisation microscope, the collagen displays a positive birefringence, the sign of which may be reversed by the phenol reaction (François et al., 1972a, 1972b and 1972c; Romhányi et al., 1973).

The reticulin consists of fine ramified fibres which are not stained by the Van Gieson method, but which are stained dark red by the PAS, red by the sulphation metachromasia method and black by silver impregnation. Saffron colours them slightly. At the polarisation microscope (François et al., 1967), the birefringence is weak, but its characteristics are the same as those of the collagen. In this case, it is necessary to use compensators or the red plate I, in order to increase the birefringence and to render it visible. In fact, from the physical point of view, between the collagen fibre and the reticulin fibre, there is only a difference of thickness and arrangement, the collagen fibrils being grouped in fibres, while the reticulin fibres remain isolated.

It seems that the reticulin constitutes a younger collagen, in fact the precursor of the adult collagen. This problem has been discussed by Seifter et al. (1968), Pearse (1972), Fraser et al. (1973).

To sum up, the definition of the term 'reticulin' is histological, in the absence of any chemical or biophysical base for differentiating it from collagen.

29

Reticulin-positive material is to be found in the activated keratocytes, but it is impossible to affirm with certitude that it is collagen. The topographical distribution of the reticulin-positive zones of the keratocytes in tissue culture nevertheless corresponds to fibrillogenetic zones described in the cornea by Payrau et al. (1967) and in other fibroblasts by Fitton-Jackson (1957, 1964).

C) Lysosomes

The lysosomes are the cellular particles discovered by De Duve and his co-workers in 1949 (De Duve, 1973). A fundamental characteristic of the lysosomes is the fact that they are surrounded by an isolating membrane. Their contents have a much more acid pH (less than 5) than the other parts of the cell. They consist of enzymes capable of catabolising (i) proteins, (ii) certain lipids and (iii) carbohydrates.

At the electron microscope, the lysosomes appear as vacuoles surrounded by a membrane and having contents of varying densities.

The lysosomes are individualised, from both the histochemical and cytochemical points of view, by the presence of acid phosphatases, which are considered as lysosomal markers.

The catabolism of the mucopolysaccharides can occur as well in the cell as at the level of the matrix, thanks to the enzymes synthesised by the reticulo-endoplasmic system. These enzymes are next surrounded by a membrane, which is formed by the Golgi's apparatus. The catabolic enzymes enclosed within a membrane constitute a primary lysosome. The fusion of a primary lysosome and a granule containing the mucopolysaccharides, or another substance to be catabolised, gives rise to a secondary lysosome. After the digestion, the content of the secondary lysosome remains in the cell (dense body), or it may be expulsed from the cell. Thanks to this process, termed exocytosis, the enzymes of the primary lysosome can also leave the cell (Fig. 7).

In that way, the dynamic equilibrium is maintained in the cell as well as in the ground substance.

The essential functions of the lysosomes are the following:
1) They are responsible for the cell autophagy.
2) They are capable of digesting phagocytosed particles. It is so that bacteria can be destroyed or isolated.
3) They play a part in the lysis process, which explains the metamorphosis of certain animals.
4) They play a part in the fertilisation process.
5) They regulate the dynamic equilibrium of the macromolecules.
6) They play a fundamental part in the cellular division and in the cell canceration.

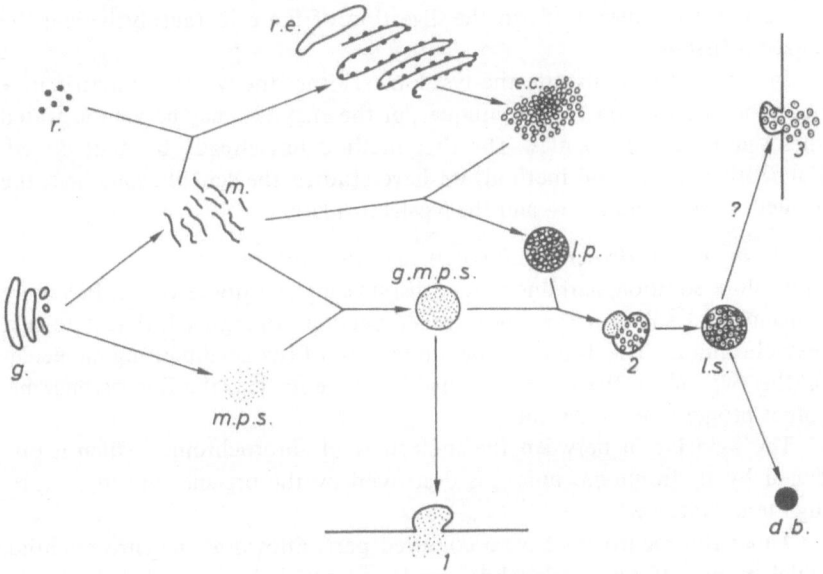

Fig. 7. Biosynthesis of the mucopolysaccharides. The Golgi's apparatus (g.) produces the membranes (m.) and synthesises the mucopolysaccharides (m.p.s.). In this manner, a mucopolysaccharide granule (g.m.p.s.) is formed. The ribosomes (r.) and the membranes (m.) form the ribosomal endoplasmic reticulum (r.e.), which synthesises the lysosomal enzymes (e.c.). These are enclosed in a membrane (m.) to form a primary lysosome (l.p.). By fusion (2) of a primary lysosome (l.p.) with a mucopolysaccharide granule (g.m.p.s.), a secondary lysosome (l.s.) is formed. This can be expelled or remain as a 'dense body' (d.b.) after intralysosomal digestion. The mucopolysaccharides can also be secreted from granules (g.m.p.s.) and expelled from the cells by exocytosis (1).

After ultracentrifuging cellular fractions, the lysosomal enzymes are inactive until they have passed through the barrier constituted by the lysosomal membrane. This is the reason why there is a latency period before their action becomes manifest.

Some enzymes that act on the mucopolysaccharides have been described: d-glucose, β-N-acetylglucosaminidase, β-glucuronidase, β-galactosidase, α-mannosidase, β-xilisidase, arylsuphatase, hyaluronidase and neuraminidase.

The most complete information about the lysosomes was given by Dingle (1972) and Dingle et al. (1973b). A description of the action of the lysosomal enzymes on hyaluronic acid was given by Morrison (1970). The histochemistry of the lysosomal system has been studied by Straus (1967) and Pearse (1972).

An insufficience of one or more lysosomal enzymes produces, in the cells and the tissues, storage of the products which should normally have been catabolised. The liberation of the enzymes, which should normally remain inside the lysosomes, leads to the digestion of the cells (autolysis) and the adjacent tissues.

In order to demonstrate the lysosomes, either the lysosomal matrix may be stained by the 'in vitro' techniques, or the enzymes may be demonstrated enclosed in the lysosomes. The first method has already been described. Concerning the second method, we have studied the acid phosphatases, the β-glucuronidase and the α- and the β-galactosidase.

Mechanism of the vital staining by acridine orange

In a dilute solution, acridine orange displays a green fluorescence. In a more concentrated solution the fluorescence becomes orange-red, that is to say, metachromatic. This is due to the interaction of the neighbouring molecules of the dye. When the solution is highly concentrated, the fluorescence becomes progressively indefinite.

The association between the molecules of fluorochrome, which is produced by hydrophobic union, is destroyed by the organic solvents and by high temperature.

Those fluorochromes have a coloured part, known as the chromophore, which is ionised and hydrophilic, and a hydrophobic part, known as the auxochrome, which is aromatic. It is this latter part which can associate with its neighbouring homologues and produce the orange-red metachromasia (Fig. 8).

Thanks to the positive charges of the chromophore, the basic dyes can associate with a polyanion. In the case of acridine orange, the polyanion may be one of the following:

1. A polysaccharide chain, which contains molecules of uronic acid and the acid groups of which are ionised as a function of the length of the polymer and the pH value of the medium. Those ionised groups must be distributed in a periodic fashion along the chain. This is the case of the acid mucopolysaccharides, which can increase their negative charges by virtue of the presence of the sulphated groups (Saunders, 1964).

2. Phospholipids, the periodic-acid groups of which are provided by the phosphated ions and the carboxyl (Barrett et al., 1968).

3. Nucleic acids (Mortelmans and Sebruyns, 1962).

When staining is effected by acridine orange or another cationic fluorochrome of the same family, unions of two types can occur:

a) A union between the negative charges of the polyanion and the positive charges of the dye. This union, which is of the electrostatic type, is brought about by coulomb attraction between the anion and the cation. It gives rise to a *green fluorescence*. It is a saline union between oppositely charged ions.

b) If the acid groups of the polyanion, to which the molecules of the dye are attached, are sufficiently abundant, an interaction will occur between the auxochrome parts of the molecules of the dye. When that union, which is of the hydrophobic type, occurs, the complex formed as a result displays a fluorescence ranging from orange to red.

There exists also an intermediate, that is to say, yellow flurorescence, when the interaction between the molecules of the dye is insufficient.

When the polyanion is highly polymerised and when its negative charges are widely spaced, the fluorochrome attached to it will give an intense green fluorescence. When the polyanion is highly polymerised and when its negative charges are very close together, the fluorescence will be an intense red.

With regard to the penetration of the dye into the cell, two mechanisms may be postulated. First, the passage of cationic substances, which depends on the energy, can take place through the cellular membrane. It is possible, indeed, to observe, at the very beginning of the staining, a green fluorescence of low intensity. Moreover, the acridine orange can pass passively through the lysosomal membrane (Barrett et al., 1968; Dingle et al., 1973a). Thinès-Sempoux (1968, 1973) showed, in addition, that there is a great similarity between the lysosomal membrane and the cellular membrane. Consequently, there is no reason why acridine orange should be able to pass through one of them and not through the other.

The other mechanism is endocytosis, by virtue of which the dye, after having been enclosed in the cell membrane (pinocytosis, vacuole), comes in contact with the primary lysosomes, which then fuse with the pinocytosis vacuoles. Indeed, peripheral vacuoles enclosing the dye may be seen. Furthermore, according to our experience, the dye diluted in the culture medium forms a colloidal solution, as we have noticed, when attempting to filter it by means of a filter having pores of from 0.2 to 0.3 μm; all the dye was

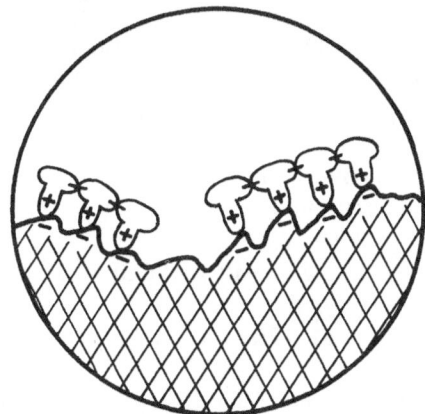

Fig. 8. The lysosomal matrix (shown cross-ruled) with its negative charges. The positive charges of the acridine orange molecules are linked to the matrix by electrostatic bonds, whereas its auxochromic groups are linked to each other to form a polymerised network.

retained by the filter. We know, moreover, that colloidal particles stimulate endocytosis and that the latter depends on energy.

Lysosomal enzymes

The *phosphatases* are the most widely distributed enzymes in the organism. They act on the phosphate esters. The *acid phosphatases* are active at lower values of pH (less than 5) than the *alkaline phosphatases*.

The substrate of the acid phosphatases is β-glycerophosphate, whereas that of the alkaline phosphatase is α-glycerophosphate (Pearse, 1972).

The acid phosphatases are exclusively lysosomal enzymes, of which they constitute effective markers.

β-glucuronidase is a lysosomal enzyme belonging to the group of hydrolases of the polysaccharides. This enzyme depolymerises the mucopolysaccharides by its action on the β-glycoside unions and contributes in that manner to the maintenance of the turn-over of the mucopolysaccharides.

Apart from the method which we have described, a new technique renders it possible to avoid the precipitates and gives more distinct positivities. It is the semipermeable-membrane method introduced by Lojda (1973 and 1974). This technique has already been applied to normal and wounded corneas with excellent results (Čejkova et al., 1975a and 1975b).

α-galactosidase and β-galactosidase are also hydrolytic enzymes acting respectively on the α- and the β-galactosides. They can also act on lactose, and for that reason, they are termed lactases. They are found in the connective and epithelial tissues, as well as in numerous bacteria (Pearse, 1972). The semipermeable-membrane method can be applied also to these enzymes.

D) Mitochondria

The mitochondria can be localised by the acridine-orange method *'in vitro'*, as we have just described. Those organelles display then a green induced fluorescence. They may also be localised by Janus green (Pearse, 1972).

We have tested two mitochondrial enzymes: glucose-6-phosphate dehydrogenase and lactic dehydrogenase. The application of these techniques to the cornea has been discussed by François et al. (1977).

IV. MICROSCOPY

a) Clear-Field microscopy

We used 'Leitz' Orthoplan and 'Zeiss' Ultraphot II microscopes.

b) Phase-contrast microscopy

We examined all our fresh and stained preparations by Zernicke's phase

34

contrast, mounted in Wild and Leitz (Orthoplan) microscopes. We also made some observations using Nomarski's interference phase-contrast technique.

c) *Dark-Field microscopy*

We used Wild and Leitz immersion condensers, as well as the Leitz dry condenser.

d) *Fluorescence microscopy*

For the various preparations treated by the several acridine-orange methods, we used the Wild fluorescence equipment and the following filters: (i) BG 12 4 mm excitation filter, which emits at wavelength 400 nm, (ii) BG38 excitation filter, emitting on 450 nm, and (iii) as stop-filter we used the orange-yellow OG 1. All the observations were made in the dark-room.

e) *Polarisation microscopy and topo-optical stainings*

We used the technique recommended by François et al. (1972a, 1972b, 1972c). We measured the birefringence with a Brace-Kohler rotatory compensator under monochromatic light ($\lambda = 580$ nm).

We studied the metachromasia with toluidine blue, the phenol reaction for changing the sign of the collagen birefringence and the rivanol staining (François et al., 1972a, 1972b, 1972c).

f) *Electron microscopy*

We fixed the specimens with glutaraldehyde and with osmic acid, buffered with 0.2M phosphate of pH 7.2. The thin sections were prepared with the aid of the Reichert ultramicrotome. They were studied at the 'Philips' electron-microscope type EM 300.

For the electron microscopy of the cells in culture, we used two methods:

1) We grew the cells on a plastics support, which we cut up. The dehydration and inclusion were effected as for an ordinary specimen.

2) Trypsinisation of a very large number of cells which are fixed and dehydrated in suspension. This treatment requires centrifuging at 700 RPM for ten minutes after each dehydrating bath. After the last bath, the Epon containing the accelerator is added, and it is polymerised. After hardening the tube is broken. In this manner, an inclusion having the same shape as the tube is obtained.

g) *Scanning microscopy*

We used the critical-point drying method recommended by Anderson (1966) and Mareel (1976). This method was adopted also, both for the histological specimens and for the monolayers. We made our observations at the Cambridge Stereoscan scanning microscope.

h) *Microcinematography*

We used the Wild equipment. The lighting was regulated so that the time of exposure of each frame was one second. The Interval between two successive frames was variable, but most commonly between fifteen and thirty seconds.

V. PHOTOGRAPHY

We used the following films:
1) Kodak Plus X-Pan for the black-and-white microphotography.
2) Kodachrome II Professional for the colour microphotography under normal lighting and at the polarisation or phase-contrast microscope.
3) Kodak High-Speed Ektachrome (daylight) for the Dark-Field and fluorescence microscopy.
4) Ilford Pan F for the black-and-white microcinematography.
5) Kodachrome 40 (Color movie film type A) for the colour microcinematography.

CHAPTER II

NORMAL KERATOCYTES 'IN SITU'

I. INTRODUCTION

According to Duke-Elder (1961), the keratocytes were described for the first time by Toynbee in 1841. Later, in 1910, Virchow called them 'corneal corpuscles'. They are practically inactive cells, which nevertheless possess all the genetic potential needed to become active in case of necessity.

Staining with silver salts has given a fairly precise idea of their shape and distribution (Krwawicz, 1947; Prieto Diaz, 1947 a and b; Sverdlick, 1954; Scharenberg, 1955; Wolter, 1957, 1959).

Jackus (1961, 1962) described them at the electron microscope. Finally, François et al. (1972c) investigated the macromolecular structure of the keratocytes 'in situ' and compared them with the fibrocytes of the sclera.

In view of the fact that the keratocytes 'in situ' have little cytoplasmic organelles capable of giving positive histochemical reactions, their study will be limited to that of the nucleus and the cell membrane.

II. PERSONAL RESULTS

a) The *phase-contrast microscope* made it possible to see, in fresh transverse sections, hydrated or dehydrated, fusiform figures located between the lamellae and corresponding to the nucleus, the cell membrane merging between the collagen lamellae. The thickness of the nuclei was from 2 to 3 μm, and their greatest length, which probably corresponded to their real length in the cell, was from 10 to 15 μm. The shorter lengths of from 5 to 10 μm doubtless corresponded to parasagital sections of the cell. The colour of the nucleus was greyish and contrasted little with the neighbouring lamellae.

b) At the *dark field microscope*, the lamellae were visible as brilliant ribbons, composed of a fine punctuation. When fresh sections or sections stained by nuclear dyes such as haematoxylin or Fast Red were examined, the cell appeared optically empty at the dark field microscope. In some cases, however, it was possible to see two or three bright spots, which corresponded to the nucleoli of the nucleus.

c) *Microscopy of stained sections under normal illumination.* – As Table II shows, most of the dyes stained the nucleus, but the staining of the cytoplasm

Table 2. Histochemistry of the normal cornea (keratocytes).

Method	Cytoplasm (granules)	Nucleus	Stroma
Haematoxilin-eosin-saffron	invisible	basophilia	yellow
Van Gieson	invisible	basophilia	red
Reticulin	–	–	++
Metachromatic curve	metachromasia between pH 2 and pH 7.6. Maximum at pH 4.9	red	metachromasia between pH 4 pH 7. Maximum between pH 5.2 and pH 6
Colloidal iron	+	red	red
Alcian blue, pH 1	+	red	+
Alcian blue, pH 2.5	+	red	+
Alcian blue, pH 6	+	red	+
Direct Schiff	–	–	–
PAS	+	–	+
Feulgen reaction	–	+	–
Acridine orange	–	green fluorescence	–
Polarisation microscopy	The keratocytes show negative birefringence		positive birefringence
Hyaluronidase test	–	[Method inapplicable]	–
Acid phosphatases	–	–	–

–Negative   +Weakly positive   ++Positive   [ ] Method inapplicable

merged with that of the neighbouring lamellae. We obtained the following results for fixed corneas:

1) With haematoxylin-eosin, the nuclei of the keratocytes took on a violet-blue colour. It was rarely possible to differentiate the nucleoli. On flat sections, one saw rounded or irregular bodies, blue in colour, which corresponded to the nuclei (Fig. 9).

2) With ferric haematoxylin, the same appearance resulted, except that the staining was brown. The nucleoli, one to three in each cell, were more easily visible. These nucleoli were also visible in the flat sections.

3) With toluidine blue, the nuclei were stained a violet-blue, that is to say, that they displayed a weak metachromasia (α-metachromasia). In the flat sections, the nucleoli could be seen displaying a stronger but heterogeneous metachromasia. The pH values that were most favourable for obtaining metachromasia were greater than 3.5; pH values of less than 3.5 gave an orthochromatic staining.

4) The direct Schiff reaction was negative.

5) On flat sections stained with PAS, more positive zones could be seen around the nucleus, which was counterstained by haematoxylin. It was, however, not possible to affirm that the cytoplasm was PAS-positive.

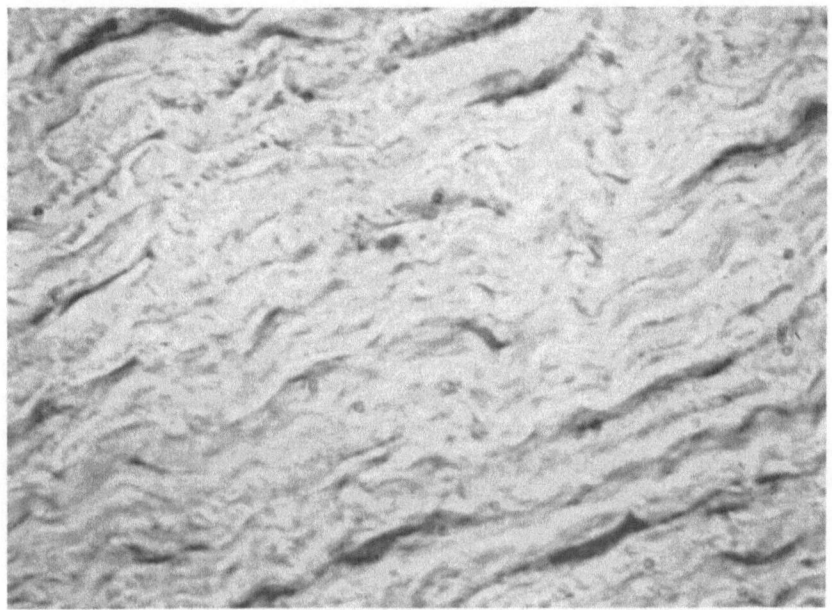

Fig. 9. Normal keratocytes *'in situ'.* Haematoxylin-eosin (x 40 obj.).

6) The most demonstrative staining was that by acridine orange, which showed the nuclei filled with DNA. The cytoplasm became positive for RNA only when the keratocyte was activated, as we shall see in Chapters IV and V. The green fluorescence filled the nucleus, which followed the often very undulating path of the lamellae immediately below and above it.

7) The staining for acid phosphatase was normally negative.

d) *Clear-Field microscopy under normal illumination of sections stained by silver nitrate.* — The best observations were given by flat and relatively thick (about 15 μm) sections. The keratocytes were arranged parallel to the surface of the cornea; they were polygonal in shape, with large pseudopodia, which gave the whole cell a star-shaped appearance. These pseudopodia were rectilinear and took up directions perpendicular to the cell body. They were in many cases bifurcated or trifurcated. These pseudopodia connected with those of the nearby keratocytes, in such a way that the cells as a whole constituted a syncytium. The area occupied by the cellular network was very large; each cellular body measured on an average from 25 to 40 μm.

The cytoplasm of the keratocytes was flattened by following the surface of the adjacent lamellae. The cytoplasmic contents were finely granulated. The edges were in many cases difficult to distinguish precisely. In some cases, very fine lines were to be seen; they crossed the cytoplasm and were probably tonofibrils.

The nucleus was eccentric in most of the cells. The irregular distribution of the chromatin gave it a pseudovesicular appearance. The nucleoli were well-defined; they numbered from one to three, and they were rounded in shape.

A similar appearance could be observed after impregnation with gold salts.

e) *Polarisation microscopy*. – We were able to confirm the results of François et al. (1972c). Polarisation microscopy using topo-optical stainings is the best method of studying the cell membrane of the keratocyte, which, with other methods, is masked by the neighbouring lamellae.

1) *Study of unstained sections mounted in arabic gum.* The membranes of the keratocytes were more birefringent than the adjacent collagen. They followed an undulating path between the lamellae. The birefringence was more accentuated at the level of the nucleus. Some of these undulating membranes extended into contiguous cells. The sign of the birefringence was negative relative to the cell surface.

After extraction of the lipids by organic solvents, the birefringence of the keratocytes disappeared.

When fresh sections in physiological saline were examined alternately at the phase-contrast microscope and at the polarisation microscope, it was seen that the keratocytes observed by phase-contrast were birefringent at the polarisation microscope, but that their birefrigence was similar to that of the lamellae. As a consequence, it was not possible to differentiate the keratocytes from the adjacent collagen. If, then, an organic solvent was applied, the birefringence of the keratocytes was seen progressively to disappear, and the keratocytes showed up as wavy black lines between the birefringent lamellae. If, next, the phase-contrast microscope was again used, the keratocytes would be found again, with the same characteristics as when first examined with that microscope.

2) *Study of fresh sections stained with topo-optical dyes.* The birefringence of the cell membrane of the keratocytes was increased by rivanol and by toluidine blue. After staining with rivanol the birefringence was six times higher than that of the unstained sections. After staining with toluidine blue, it was four times higher. Azur A gave the same result as toluidine blue.

The intrinsic birefringence always remained negative after topo-optical staining.

In the stained sections, the cell membranes absorbed only light polarised perpendicularly to the cell surface. There was no absorption when the light was polarised longitudinally relative to the cell surface.

After extraction of the lipids and staining with toluidine blue, the birefringence of the membranes disappeared, but on normal microscopical examination, it was seen that the staining persisted, which implied that the lipids oriented the molecules of the dye, but did not themselves become stained.

When a metachromasia curve for toluidine was drawn, it could be seen that the birefringence was present, although weak, for pH values less than 3. For pH values between 3 and 4, it increased suddenly, but there was no further increase for pH values higher than 4.

These changes in the birefringence occurred at the same pH as that of the mucopolysaccharides oriented along the collagen fibres of the stroma.

f) *Electron microscopy of the keratocytes 'in situ'.* – At the electron microscope, the keratocytes *'in situ'* displayed the characteristics of inactive cells:

1). The nucleus had a granular and dense chromatin, which contained nucleoli of heterogeneous electron density.

2). The nuclear membrane was well defined and constituted a membrane unit having two electron-dense bands, with a light area between them; these were the two protein layers, the central lipid area having been removed by the dehydration process and as a consequence being electronically empty.

3). An area of greater electron density was observed against the internal proteinic layer of the nuclear membrane.

4). The lighter cytoplasm was represented by a finely granulated matrix.

5) There were only very few intra-cytoplasmic organelles. Some mitochondria or vacuoles – in many cases empty and surrounded by a membrane – were seen.

6). The cell membrane constituted also a membrane unit, having characteristics similar to those of the nuclear membrane.

The distance between the protein layers was 120 Å.

The nuclear membrane was closely surrounded by the matrix of the ground substance of the stroma. The first collagen fibres had very uniform diameters.

DISCUSSION AND CONCLUSIONS

In the keratocytes *in situ*, the most noteworthy structures are the nucleus and the cytoplasmic membrane.

The nucleus takes on positive staining with all the usual nuclear dyes. It contains one to three nucleoli, which consist of a substance of heterogeneous electron density.

The nucleus displays a green fluorescence after fixation and staining with acridine orange, which indicates the presence of DNA.

We were not able, by this method, to identify RNA in the cytoplasm.

As a whole, the cell is flattened between the lamellae and conforms with their undulations.

Sections stained by silver impregnation (Krwawicz, 1947; Prieto Diaz,

1947a and b; Sverdlick, 1954; Scharenberg, 1955; Wolter, 1957, 1959; Duke-Elder, 1961; personal observation) show that the mass of cells arranges itself as a syncytium, thanks to the intertwining pseudopodia. This method shows up the cytoplasm and the nuclei.

The measurement of transverse sections at the electron microscope shows that the thickness of the cells is 2 μm (Scorcia, 1973).

The methods that give most information about the cytoplasmic membrane are polarisation microscopy (François et al., 1972b; personal observation) and electron microscopy. The intrinsic negative birefringence of the membrane is due to the lipid structures oriented perpendicularly to the membrane surface. This birefringence is similar to that of other fibrocytes and corresponds perfectly to that of the membranes of cultivated keratocytes.

The lipids of the membranes of the keratocytes are similar to those of other cells, such as the fibrocytes of the sclera or the endothelial cells of the cornea, although their structure is different from that of myelin and of external segments of photoreceptors (François et al., 1972b; personal observation).

The increase of the birefringence is due to the fact that the molecules of dye orient themselves on the membrane, adding their own refringence to that of the cell.

The following are the conclusions of François et al. (1972b) concerning the topo-optical stainings:

1. The cellular membrane absorbs light polarised perpendicularly to the membrane, but not that which is polarised longitudinally to it.

2. The absorption is a maximum for the green colour.

3. The changes of anisotropy and dichroism prove that the cationic dyes are linked perpendicularly to the cellular surface.

4. The fact that the birefringence due to topo-optical dyes disappears after extraction of the fats, although the staining itself is not eliminated (it remains still visible by clear-field microscopy) proves that the dye is oriented by the lipid layer of the membrane. It is not, however, the lipids themselves that are stained, it is rather the polysaccharides linked to the membrane (glycocalix).

The birefringence due to toluidine blue is still present at pH of less than 3, which indicates the ionisation of acid groups of low pH values.

The metachromatic curves and that of birefringence coincide, for by clear-field microscopy metachromasia at a pH less than 3 is also found in the zone, which corresponds to the keratocyte membrane. All these facts argue in favour of the presence of highly negatively ionised molecules linked to the surface of the cellular membrane.

The collagen of the neighbouring corneal stroma displays, moreover, a positive intrinsic birefringence, since the semi-crystals of tropo-collagen are arranged longitudinally in the fibres and since the mucopolysaccharides which are linked to it display the same characteristics as those that are linked to the keratocyte membrane. In addition, the molecules of kerato-sulphate also are oriented perpendicularly to the collagen fibre, as their intrinsic birefringence is negative.

The distance between the molecules of toluidine blue must be 5 Å, if the auxochrome groups of the dye (colourless aromatic groups of the dye) are to be able to link together laterally, producing thereby a metachromatic staining as we described before. In that case, in view of the fact that the structure is periodic (-dye-mucopolysaccharide-dye-mucopolysaccharide-), it may be assumed that the molecules of mucopolysaccharides are themselves also spaced at distance of 5 Å one from another.

The electron microscope shows the *membrane unit*. After the extraction of the lipids, the cell membrane displays two layers of high electron density, formed by the proteins. The central light band represents the place where the molecules of lipids were arranged perpendicularly.

Fig. 10 shows the structure of the macromolecular complex formed by the collagen containing the kerato-sulphate and the keratocyte membrane.

According to François et al. (1972b), the lipid layer of loose structure is probably composed of phospholipids and unsaturated chains of hydrocarbons.

According to Danielli's model, the hydrophobic groups of the lipid chains are polarised toward the proteinic layers, whereas the hydrophilic poles are face to face (Fig. 10).

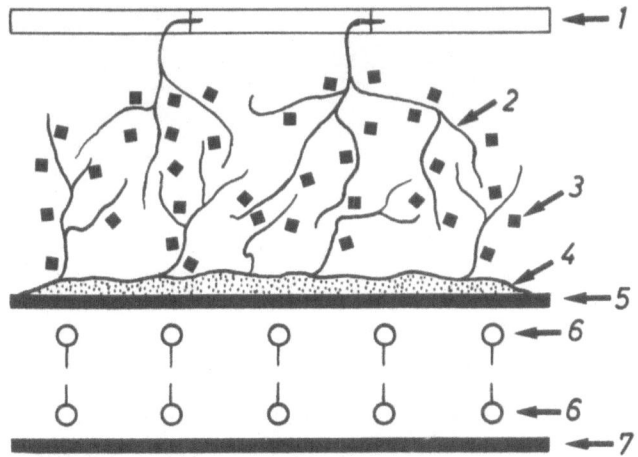

Fig. 10. Probable relationship between the keratocyte membrane and the surrounding stroma: 1. fibrillar protein (collagen); 2. mucopolysaccharide chains; 3. molecules of water; 4. mucopolysaccharide chains of the cellular surface; 5. external protein layer of the keratocyte cytoplasmic membrane unit; 6. lipid layers; 7. internal protein layer.

The proteins are probably arranged in the form of a molecular film.

The cytoplasmic matrix is excessively poor in organelles, with the result that it may be considered to be inactive. Nevertheless, Scorcia (1973) in many cases found a Golgi's apparatus.

In the corneas of children, on the other hand, active cells containing large numbers of organelles can be found. However, what above all characterises these cells is the presence of an electron-dense and finely granulated substance, which accumulates against the cell membrane and can sometimes deform the nucleus (Payrau et al., 1967). That material has been observed also in keratoconus (Jackus, 1961 and 1962; Payrau et al., 1967; Hamada et al., 1972). These areas are similar to those described by Fitton-Jackson (1964), during the fibrillogenesis of collagen in the fibroblasts.

In conclusion, the keratocyte *'in situ'* of the adult is a practically inactive cell having a very developed cellular membrane which forms a syncytium. These cells nevertheless have the genetic potential needed for their activation and their proliferation. The cellular membrane and the tonofibrils enable the cell to spread between the collagen lamellae of the stroma and, in tissue culture, to migrate on the walls of the culture flask.

CHAPTER III

ARCHITECTONIC OF THE CORNEA

I. INTRODUCTION

The normal keratocytes, which we have studied in the preceding Chapter, are distributed between the corneal lamellae. These lamellae have a most particular architectonic, which determines the form and the distribution of the keratocytes *in situ*. For that reason, we shall describe the microscopical appearance of the corneal stroma, and present an architectonic interpretation of it.

The structure of the stroma is extremely important, because the collagen and the mucopolysaccharides, which display a very regular arrangement, are formed by the keratocytes during the embryonic development and early infancy.

The constituent elements of the cornea have well proportioned dimensions. Histological studies using optical and electron microscopes, the silver impregnation methods and the optical properties of the cornea make it possible to determine its architectonic, as well as the stabilising factors.

While studying the collagen fascicles at the electron microscope, Jackus (1961) found that they crossed one to another at right angles. That fact was the starting point of our topographical study of the corneal stroma.

II. PERSONAL RESULTS

We shall describe successively the anterior central part, the posterior central part, the intermediate zone between the central and peripheral parts, as well as the periphery of the cornea.

In situ, the greatest concentration of keratocytes is found in the central part. In the corneal periphery, the cell population is heterogeneous, since fibroblasts and mast cells are also found there.

A. Flat sections

1) *Anterior central part.* — At the phase-contrast microscope, the corneal fascicles had widths of 10 to 20 μm; their lengths were extremely variable. They crossed one another at very different angles, even those fascicles that were in exactly the same plane. Each fascicle could align itself obliquely from the surface toward the depth of the lamella.

At the electron microscope, the interfascicular angles were irregular, al-

12 h

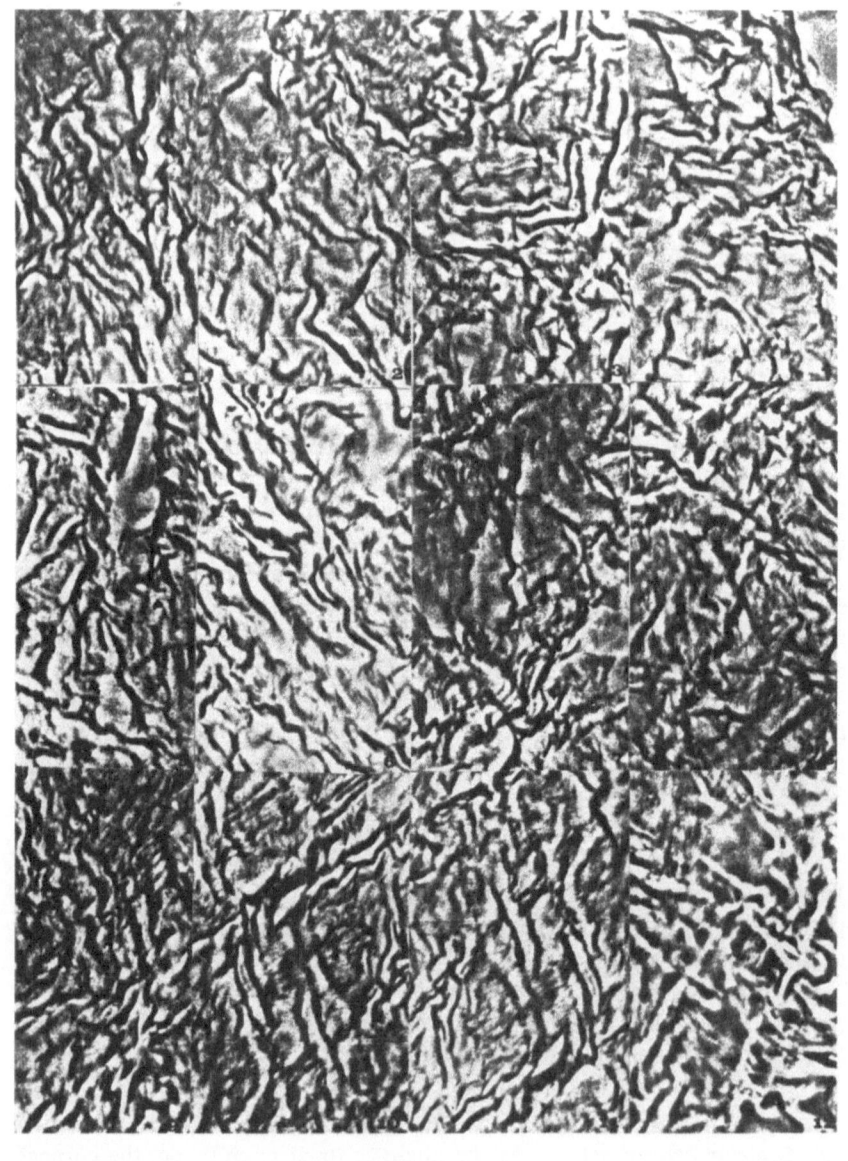

9 h

3 h

6 h

Fig. 11. Collagen fascicles in the posterior central part of the cornea. Flat sections from the surface to the depth. Sections Nos. 3, 4, 9, 10, 11 and 12 show right interfascicular angles. Phase-contrast microscopy (x 20 obj.).

46

though it was possible to find some right angles. There was no relationship between the interfascicular angles of the various planes of the same lamella.

2) *Posterior central part* — Here the fascicles were easier to follow, but their dimensions were the same as those of the anterior part (Fig. 11).

When 3-μm sections were examined, a large number of fascicles was found, crossing one another at right angles, although, at the level of any given plane, fascicles coming from a lower or a higher plane could be found, crossing the observation field obliquely. On the whole, the appearance was rectangular.

A study of successive seriated sections showed a rotation of those rectangular figures in a clockwise sense, but an orthogonal arrangement as described by Coulombre et al. (1961) was not seen.

Before the Descemet's membrane, the arrangement became irregular.

At the electron microscope, most of the interfascicular angles were right.

3) *Intermediate part.* — In the depth of the stroma, we found an arrangement similar to that of the posterior central part.

4) *Periphery of the cornea.* — The fascicles became irregular and bifurcated. In addition, a large quantity of circular fibres was found (Fig. 12).

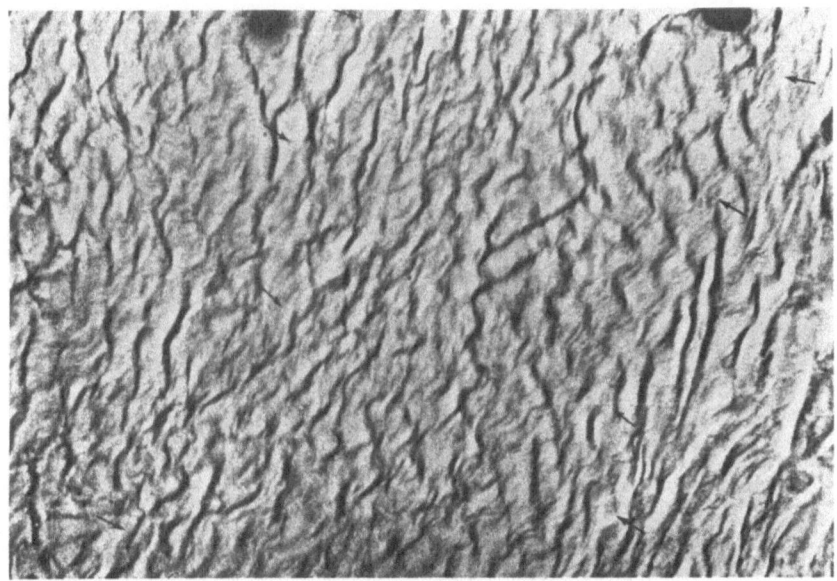

Fig. 12. Seriated sections of the corneal periphery. The arrows indicate Polack's circular fascicle. Phase-contrast microscopy (x 20 obj.).

B. Transversal sections

It is not necessary to stress the lamellar structure of the cornea, the regularity of which contrasts with that of the sclera. We nevertheless draw attention to the existence of interlamellar fascicles, which pass from one lamellar level to another after a short distance. It is these fascicles that are cut when a lamellar keratoplasty or dissection of the lamellae is performed.

At the electron microscope, the thickness of the fascicles was regular. The fibres belonging to any given plane displayed a direction either perpendicular or oblique relative to the planes above and below. The fibrils had a regular diameter and arranged themselves in a hexagonal disposition.

C. Study of flat sections at the polarisation microscope

1) *Anterior central part.* — When the collagen fascicles lied in the same plane as that of the vibration of the polarised light, they displayed a positive birefringence, whereas these which lied in a plane perpendicular to that plane showed a negative birefringence (Fig. 13).

In the anterior central part, the arrangement of the collagen fascicles was very irregular; many obliquely disposed fascicles were found.

2) *Posterior central part* (Fig. 14). — Most of the interfascicular angles were right. Some oblique fibres coming from the planes above and below

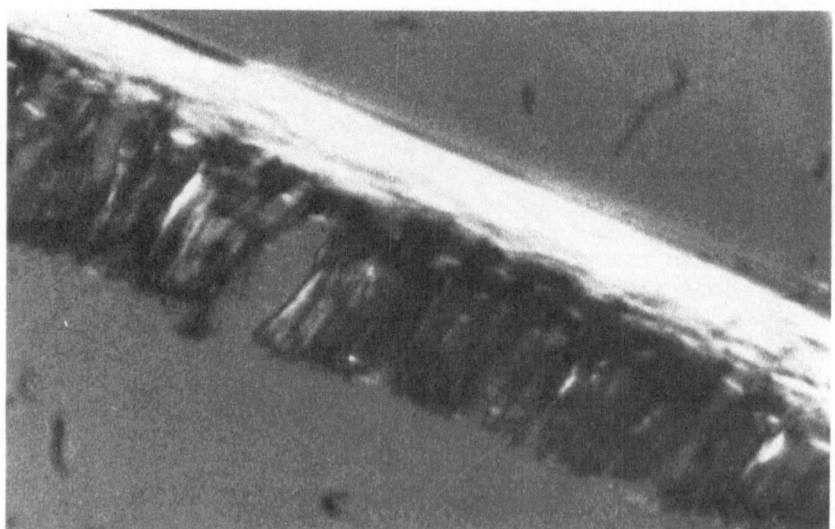

Fig. 13. Positive birefringence of a collagen fascicle and negative birefringence of the extremities of several fascicles arranged at right angles.

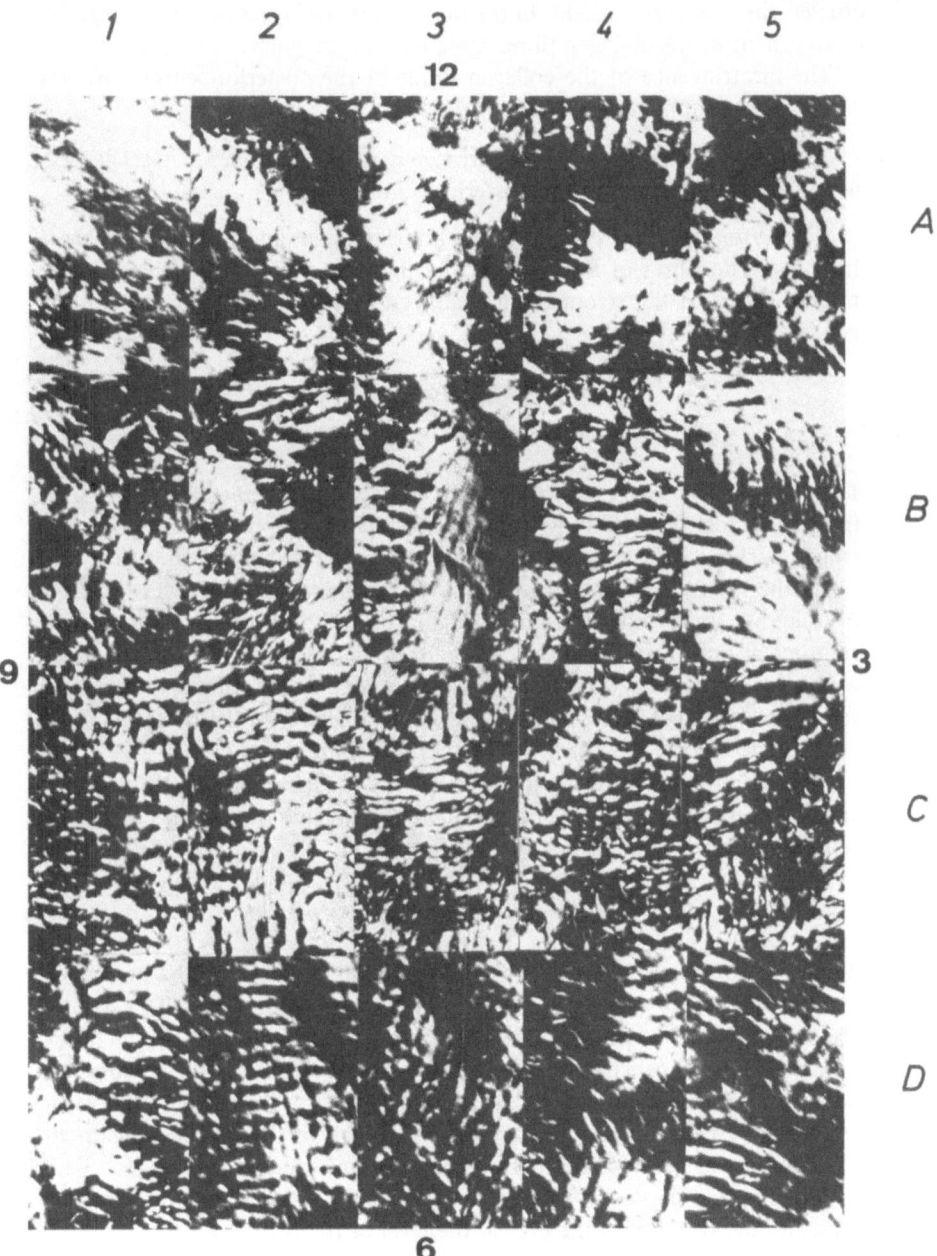

Fig. 14. Flat and seriated sections of the collagen fascicles in the central part of the cornea. Sections Nos. B3, B5, C1 to C5 and D1 to D5 show fascicles arranged at right angles. Several oblique angles are also visible. Polarisation microscopy (x 16 obj.).

crossed the observation field. In the most posterior layers of the stroma, the arrangement of the collagen fibres again became irregular.

The birefringence of the collagen fibres of the posterior central part was weaker than that of the anterior part.

3) *Intermediate part.* — The arrangement of the collagen fascicles was here identical with that of the posterior central part.

4) *Periphery of the cornea.* — The interfascicular angles were much more irregular. The fibres of Polack's circular ligament were more evident in the middle layers of the stroma, and displayed a very intense positive birefringence.

D. Study of transversal sections at the polarisation microscope

The collagen fibres were birefringent. Each lamella was formed by parallel birefringent bands, separated by dark bands, which corresponded to fascicles arranged perpendicularly to the direction of the birefringent bands (Fig. 15).

At the limbus, alongside the regular corneal lamellae, there were collagen fascicles becoming more and more irregular as the sclera was approached. The anatomical limit between the cornea and the sclera was made by a triangular wedge of the cornea, which was inset in a scleral slot matching the shape of the corneal triangle. The anterior angle was longer than the posterior angle, which ended at the level of the sclero-corneal trabeculum.

That anatomical limit, easily visible at the polarisation microscope, coincided with the limit of the corneal mucopolysaccharides, as was shown by staining with colloidal iron or Alcian blue (pH1).

E. Study of the mucopolysaccharides

When Alcian blue (pH 1 or 2.5) was used, the full thickness of the stroma was stained. The staining could be localised at the level of the fibres. This staining was in fact due to the mucopolysaccharidic sheaths around the collagen fibres.

When the corneal stroma was stained with colloidal iron, the staining was positive at the level of the collagen fibres, which were stained blue. If, in addition, Van Gieson's counter staining was used, the blue of the mucopolysaccharides was masked, all the fibres being stained red.

When PAS and saffron were used together, the staining due to the saffron masked the positivity of the PAS at the level of the fibrils.

The zone of metachromasia of the cornea extended as far as the anatomical limit. It was produced for pH values between 3.5 and 8. The metachromasia of the sclera was weaker.

In congenital oedematous dystrophy of the cornea, Victoria-Troncoso et

50

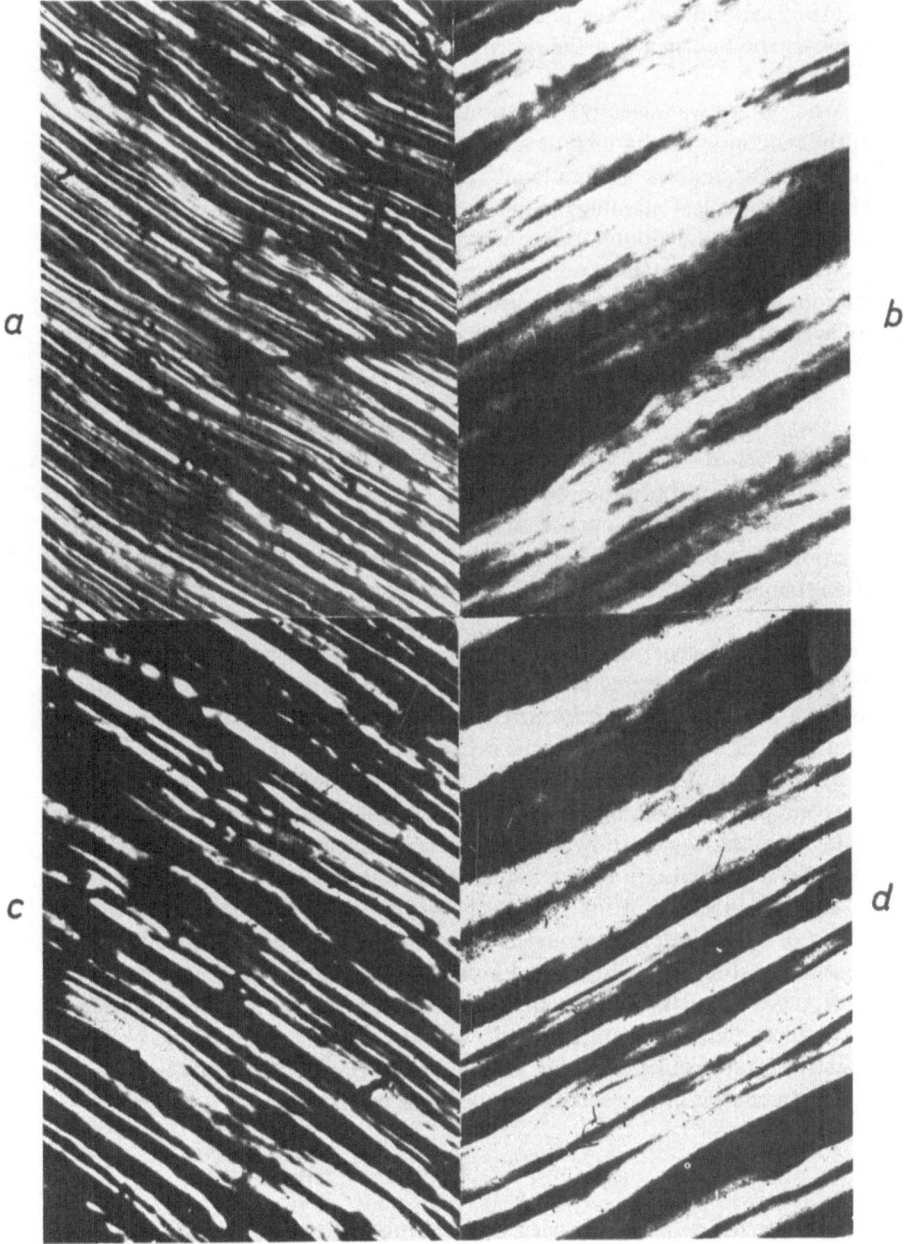

Fig. 15. Lamellae of the cornea (a) and of the sclera (b) (× 20 obj.). Lamellae of the cornea (c) and of the sclera (d) (× 100 obj.).

al. (1969) found, using the phase-contrast microscope, an optical disphasing between the collagen and the mucopolysaccharides, which seemed to form sheaths.

When there was selective digestion of the collagen without deterioration of the mucopolysaccharides, as seen in macular dystrophy of the cornea, the mucopolysaccharides accumulated freely, without linking to the collagen. The histochemical stainings made it possible to distinguish easily the collagen from the mucopolysaccharides.

When a section stained with Alcian blue was examined at the polarisation microscope, the birefringence was blue. The dye thus did not dissociate the collagen fibres from the mucopolysaccharides, the two structures constituting a single histochemical unit.

F. Topo-optical study

The topo-optical study showed:

1) When the birefringence of the collagen was reversed by the phenol reaction, a negative axial birefringence having a delay of 17 nm was observed after staining with toluidine blue. This fact indicated, on the one hand, that the molecules of the dye were arranged periodically and perpendicularly to the mucopolysaccharide chains, and, on the other hand, that the polyanionic chains were arranged parallel to the molecules of tropo-collagen, which, for their part, were arranged longitudinally relative to the collagen fibrils. The birefringence diminished with the pH of the dye and indicated a diminution in the number of free negative charges. That reduction of the birefringence between pH 4.5 and pH 1 evolved in parallel with the decrease of the metachromasia, which showed that the crystalline structure was produced by the orderly distribution of the toluidine blue molecules.

2) The blocking of the anionic charges by methylation and the neutralisation of the collagen birefringence by the phenol caused the disappearance of the metachromasia and of the birefringence of the polyanionic chains.

If, next, the dialdehyde groups were oxidised with 0.01% periodic acid and then sulphated, the metachromasia would reappear, at the same time as a negative birefringence, which confirmed the parallel arrangement of the mucopolysaccharide chains relative to the collagen fibrils.

G. Diffraction by X-rays

The collagen fibre of the cornea displayed molecules of tropo-collagen forming a semi-crystalline structure, which we examined with the wide-angle X-ray diffractometer. The essential characteristics of this structure were:

1) Two symmetrical meridional arcs spaced at 2.9Å were seen.

2) There were less intense and more diffuse reflections spaced at about 6 or 12 Å.

3) There were equatorial reflections spaced at 4.5 Å.

H. Examination of collagen-mucopolysaccharide complexes at the high-resolution electron microscope

When the collagen-mucopolysaccharide complexes were observed at the high-resolution electron microscope after staining with Alcian blue, it was seen that the mucopolysaccharides inserted themselves periodically and perpendicularly relative to the collagen fibre.

I. Macromolecular model of the corneal stroma

The tropo-collagen was arranged in fibrils. Its macromolecular organisation corresponded, according to the diffractograms, to Ramachadran's model.

As indicated in Fig. 16, the molecules of tropocollagen overlapped by a quarter of their length. The total length of the molecule was 2800 Å. The periodicity of the fibril was 2800 Å ÷ 4 ≈ 700 Å, and in fact 640 Å.

The polyanionic chains, whether or not associated with a structured protein, were inserted perpendicularly to the collagen fibril and immediately changed direction, in order to arrange themselves parallel to the fibril, with the result that the polysaccharide chains, together with the structure protein, constituted a sheath in the form of a 'pony tail' around the fibril.

The presence of numerous negative charges made possible the hydration of the stroma. The position of the water molecules is indicated in Fig. 10.

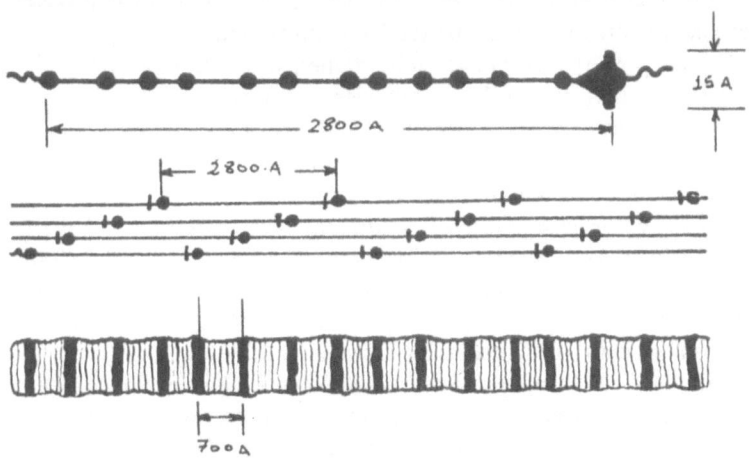

Fig. 16. Distribution of the tropocollagen molecules along the fibre.

53

The cellular membrane of the keratocytes displayed a classical arrangement with bimolecular proteinolipidic layers.

The glycocalix of the keratocytes merged with the mucopolysaccharides of the ground substance. The macromolecular model of the keratocyte is seen in Fig. 10, which was drawn on the basis of the topo-optical observations.

DISCUSSION

According to Coulombre (1957) and Coulombre et al. (1958), the normal ontogenetic development of the cornea depends above all on the tangential forces produced in the wall of the ocular globe by the expansion of the vitreous.

Those authors observed that the curvature of the cornea of the chicken embryo appears after fourteen days of incubation, immediately after the appearance of the mucopolysaccharides. In addition, the hydrophilia of the lamellae diminishes, as the age of the cornea increases.

The cornea is thinner in the centre than at its periphery. The vertical anterior radius of curvature is 7.7 mm, the horizontal anterior radius 7.8 mm, the vertical posterior radius 6.6 mm, and the horizontal posterior radius 6.22 mm. The thickness is between 0.53 and 0.54 mm at the centre and increases toward the periphery. The anterior area of the cornea is 130 mm^2. Its average diameter is 11.6 mm, the extremes being 9 and 13.5 mm. The top is 2.684 mm above the plane of the limbus (Payrau et al., 1967).

The optical methods, investigating the interference of the light (Coulombre et al., 1961) and the studies at the polarisation microscope (Naylor, 1953; François et al., 1966, 1967 and Varga et al., 1970) made it possible to determine the orientation of the fascicles and the fibres.

The study of the 10-μm sections stained with silver carbonate (Polack, 1961) shows that the collagen fascicles are irregularly distributed in the different lamellae, whereas Jackus (1954, 1961) found that the corneal fascicles joined up at right angles in the rat and in man.

In the chicken, Coulombre et al. (1961) observed an irregular arrangement of the fascicles at the level of the anterior central part of the cornea and an orthogonal arrangement elsewhere. The fascicles cross each other at right angles, and these angles rotate through 45° clockwise in each of the deeper layers. Naylor (1953), Pratt-Johnson (1959) and Polack (1961) found, on the contrary, an anarchic arrangement.

At the level of the anterior third of the central part of the cornea, which is the last to be formed embryologically, that is to say at the time of birth (Smelser et al., 1957, 1959), we found an irregular arrangement of the fascicles. At the level of the posterior third of the central and paracentral

54

parts, the fascicles that lie in the same plane cross one another at right angles, but they are at the same time crossed obliquely by fascicles coming from higher and lower planes. There exist, indeed interlamellar fascicles that pass from one layer to another.

Flat sections of the corneal periphery show circular fascicles forming a kind of circular ligament. This observation confirms those of Pratt-Johnson (1959) and Polack (1961).

The cornea is constituted of lamellae, which are formed of collagen fascicles arranged as we have just described. We were able to confirm the fact that the cornea is embedded in the sclera, the anatomical limit being marked by the presence of mucopolysaccharides, which can be demonstrated histochemically. There are, indeed, differences in the staining by pH 1 Alcian blue and in the metachromasia. The latter is more intense in the cornea, where the polyanionic surface is larger, thanks to the -SH groups of the acid mucopolysaccharides. These observations confirm those of Smelser et al. (1957, 1959), who investigated the incorporation of S^{35}.

The fascicles are constituted of collagen fibres, easily visible at the optical and polarisation microscopes. These fibres measure 0.35 μm (François et al., 1966, 1967). The collagen fibres are formed of fibrils, visible at the electron microscope. Hamada et al. (1972) found that the mean diameter of these fibrils is 225 Å, and that it increases linearly by 30 Å from the surface to the depth, without changing from the centre to the periphery. Jackus (1954, 1961) found a smaller value (190 Å) and François et al. (1953, 1954) a higher value (300-350 Å), the axial periodicity of the fibrils being 640 Å. We noted that the fibrils, which arrange themselves in a hexagonal meshwork, have diameters between 250 and 300 Å. The differences between the authors' observations depend probably on the methods of fixation, inclusion and measurement.

The collagen fibres are formed by molecules of tropocollagen, arranged parallel to the axis of the fibril, as in the other collagen tissues (Naylor, 1953; François et al., 1966, 1967; Varga et al., 1970). The periodicity found by François et al. (1953, 1954) shows that these molecules, which have a length of 2800 Å, are so arranged that the extremities of each molecule coincide with one of the quarters of the length of the adjacent molecule (2800 Å ÷ 4 ≈ 640 Å).

The molecules of kerato-sulphate, whether or not associated with molecules of non-collagen proteins, form fibrils, which have very numerous negative charges and together constitute real polyanionic surfaces.

The molecules of tropo-collagen of the neighbouring fibrils can unite by molecular condensation, to produce a miscellar structure (Naylor, 1953), which explains the association, not only between the fibrils, but also between the fascicles and the lamellae.

The properties of a given connective tissue depend upon the association

55

between the mucopolysaccharides and the collagen. As regards the cornea, the regularity of the structure is due to the presence of a particular mucopolysaccharide, namely keratosulphate, which associates with the collagen and the non collagenous structural protein.

It has been shown recently that the mucopolysaccharides can crystallise *in vitro* (Atkins et al., 1973), which makes it possible to study them with the X-ray diffractometer. As the spatial structure of the molecules can so be analysed, molecular models can be constructed. Atkins et al. (1973) constructed one for dermatan sulphate, which can have three structures (Fig. 17).

1) A helix turning to the left, each unit repeating every eighth turn of the spiral. The disaccharides repeat along an axis of 0.93 nm.

2) A helix turning to the left, each unit repeating every third turn of the spiral. The disaccharides repeat along an axis of 0.95 nm.

3) A helix turning to the left, each unit repeating every third turn of the spiral. The disaccharides repeat along an axis of 0.97 nm.

As far as we know, these observations have not been confirmed for keratosulphate, although the crystalline state has been demonstrated by François et al. (1972b).

It has, however, not been demonstrated that *in vivo* all the chains form helices.

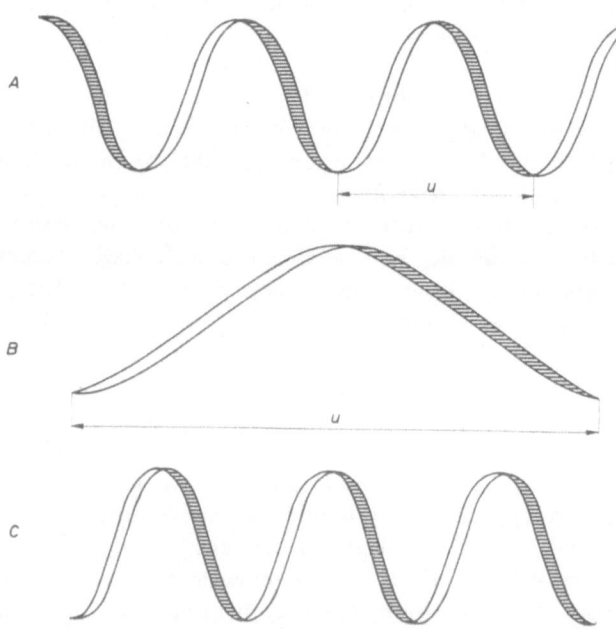

Fig. 17. The three helicoidal structures of dermatan sulphate. X-Ray diffraction study (Atkins and Isaac, 1973).

We were able to obtain diffractograms of the mucopolysaccharides of the cornea.

In vivo, the mucopolysaccharides may be found in two different forms:

1) *In the form of a ball*, the chains being rolled up on themselves. This form is encountered above all in the liquids (the synovial liquid and probably also the aqueous humour), but also in the keratocytes and the corneal stroma, in case of mucopolysaccharidosis.

2) *In a linear form.* — Over a certain part of their length, the chains would be linked to proteins and particularly to the collagen. Proteoglycans or proteino-mucopolysaccharides are so formed.

We modified the structural model of Mathews (1969, 1970), which we have already described. The diagram shows that the mucopolysaccharide chain displays a free part and a part linked to the collagen. The free part comprises a great number of free negative charges (Fig. 18), which are responsible for the positive histochemical stainings. This positivity is directly proportional to the length of the chain, and the latter depends upon the catabolic enzymes originating in the lysosomes of the keratocytes. The free part, which behaves like a free mucopolysaccharide, can attract water.

The number of chains linked to each collagen fibril is variable. In the experimental models, there is a saturation point (Mathews, 1970). The number of chains can, however, be sufficient to form a 'pony tail' or a real sleeve around each collagen fibril. We found also such sheaths around the collagen fibres of the vitreous (François et al., 1969).

A certain number of free chains can appear in the form of a helix, that is to say, in the crystalline state. They may then display phenomena of posi-

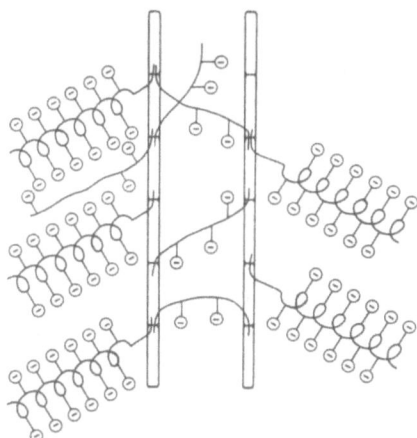

Fig. 18. Model of non-hydrated mucopolysaccharides linked to the collagen. The negative charges of the mucopolysaccharides are indicated (after Mathews, 1970, modified).

tive or negative birefringence, as we were able to observe in the cornea and the vitreous (François et al., 1966, 1967). François et al. (1972b) studied the birefringence of the corneal mucopolysaccharides, by reversing the sign of the birefringence of the collagen by the phenol reaction. Under these conditions, the mucopolysaccharides display a bright positive birefringence, whereas the collagen displays a negative birefringence in the form of black lines.

As each free chain of mucopolysaccharide carries negative charges, there is repulsion between the chains, which remain independent, and for that reason possess an electronically and biologically active surface.

Over one part of its length, the mucopolysaccharide chain remains fixed to the collagen fibril by lateral links between its own chain and that of the triple helix of the tropocollagen. These links are electrostatic and steric (Mathews, 1970).

Fig. 19 shows us the model in the hydration state, that is to say, in the state of 'biological oedema'. This increases in volume and may displace neighbouring structures.

Supplementary information can be found in the papers of Mathews (1969, 1970), Obrink (1970), Hoffman et al. (1970), Lowther et al. (1970), Serafini-Fracassini et al. (1970). The structure of hyaluronic acid was studied by Swann (1970), Laurent (1970) and Jacobson (1970).

In the case of leucoma, the regularity of the corneal architectonic is upset. It is also disturbed in the case of hydration (Smelser, 1952; Harris, 1957).

Descemet's membrane constitutes an elastic supporting ligament, the insertion of which is at the level of the scleral trabeculum.

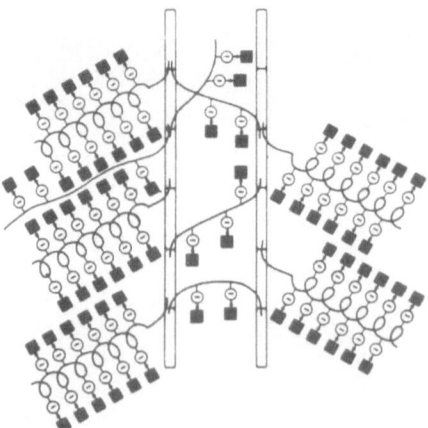

Fig. 19. Model of hydrated mucopolysaccharides linked to the collagen. The molecules of water are indicated by black squares.

Bowman's membrane is formed of fine collagen fibres (Jackus, (1961), although it normally appears to be homogeneous at the optical microscope. In certain cases, however, as in keratoconus, it may have a fibrillar appearance, even at the optical microscope.

Topo-optical stainings and examination at the electron microscope permit the following conclusions (Fig. 20 I)

1) The proteino-mucopolysaccharidic complexes are arranged parallel to the collagen fibrils.

2) These complexes have negative charges, which depend upon the sulphated and carboxyl groups, and are arranged periodically.

3) The blocking of the negative charges by methylation, and the demonstration of neighbouring hydroxyl groups, oxidised with aldehyde, confirm the parallelism between the collagen and the polysaccharidic chains.

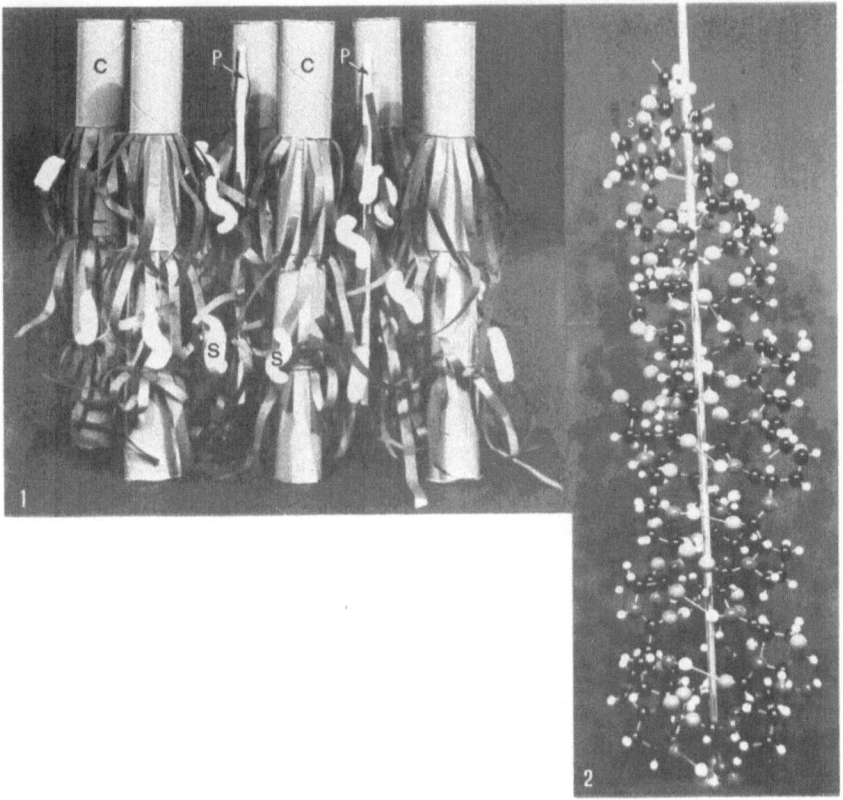

Fig. 20. I. Model showing the distribution of the corneal macromolecules. C: collagen fibrils. P: structural proteins. M: mucopolysaccharidic chains. S: soluble fraction. II. Ramachandran's model of tropocollagen.

4) The associated polysaccharidic chains are inserted perpendicularly, relative to the collagen fibril.

Diffraction with X-rays contributes in effect nothing new, as the type of the tropocollagen molecules and their arrangement are similar to those of other tissues, the architectonic regularity and the regularity of the diameters being due to the macromolecular organisation of the ground substance (Fig. 20 II).

The action of the lysosomal enzymes contained in the keratocytes activated by an infection or by a dystrophy can give rise to a cytolysis, followed by a disorganisation of the structures that surround the destroyed cell.

CHAPTER IV

THE KERATOCYTES IN THE PROCESS OF CICATRISATION OF THE CORNEAL STROMA

The object of these experiments was the investigation, from the histochemical and microscopical points of view, of the behaviour of the keratocytes in corneal wounds.

I. PERSONAL OBSERVATIONS

A. *Transformation of the keratocytes in a wound*

We studied central incisions into the cornea, because they enable to observe 'pure' keratocytes, free of contamination by other cells. We studied at the same time the culture of the keratocytes of the fellow eye, wounded in the same way.

During the first forty-eight hours, we observed histologically a drift of the epithelial cells and their proliferation in the incision wound (Fig. 21). Next, there was a proliferation of connective tissue, which pressed back the epithelial invagination (Fig. 22).

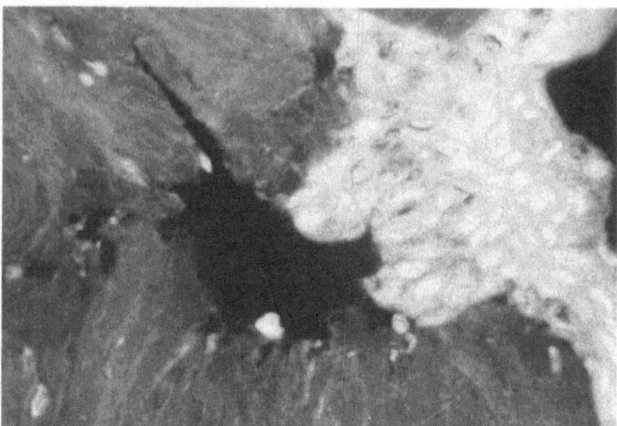

Fig. 21. An epithelial proliferation developed during the first twenty-four hours after the incision. The stroma displays inactive cells. The epithelial cells show an orange (RNA) and green (DNA) fluorescence. Acridine orange. Fluorescence microscopy (x 20 obj.).

We did not study the perforating wounds of the cornea in the rabbit. The aqueous humour of this animal contains a large quantity of fibrin, which avoids the normal contact between the lips of the wound.

The phenomena that we will describe depend exclusively on the keratocytes. Indeed, when the wound is small and central, the cornea can cicatrise in the absence of vessels, which carry other types of tissue cells.

During the first twenty-four hours, easily recognizable polynuclears, originating probably from the precorneal lacrimal film, might invade the wound. They were extremely few in number, when the operation was carried out under sterile conditions and when the incision caused only a slight traumatism. They disappeared as soon as the wound was again covered by epithelium.

During the first twenty-four hours, we observed the following morphological changes:

1. An increase in the volume and the number of nucleoli (four to five per cell), which demonstrated that the nucleus was becoming active.

2. An increase in the cytoplasmic volume, the cytoplasmic extensions becoming shorter and the cells taking on a more star-shaped appearance.

These changes did not occur in the wound itself, which was oedematous and remained free of keratocytes, but rather at a distance of 200 or 250 μm.

During this latency period, there was no cell division, although the keratocytes became active.

Twenty-four to seventy-two hours later, we observed mitoses, which reached a maximum between the third and the fifth days. Most of the cells of the central corneal wounds originated from the division of keratocytes. These contained keratosulphate granules, which made it possible to identify

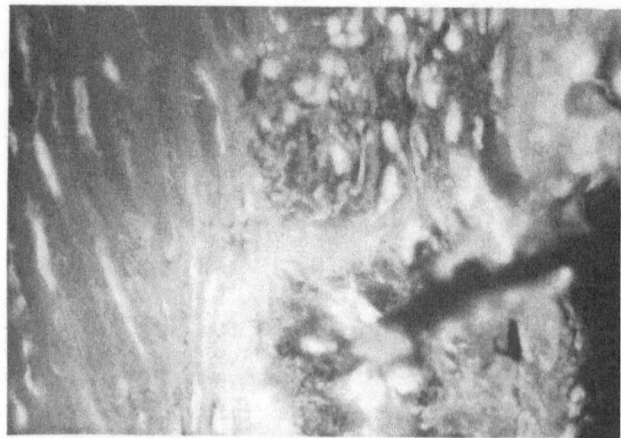

Fig. 22. After seventy-two hours numerous keratocytes have proliferated. They show a red fluorescence (RNA). Acridine orange. Fluorescence microscopy (x 10 obj.).

them. In our experiments on the rabbit cornea, we found that 90% of the cells contained keratosulphate.

The keratocytes remained unchanged morphologically between the fifth and the fifteenth day. From the fifteenth day onward, their number decreased. Between the first and the third month, the cytoplasm and the nucleus regressed.

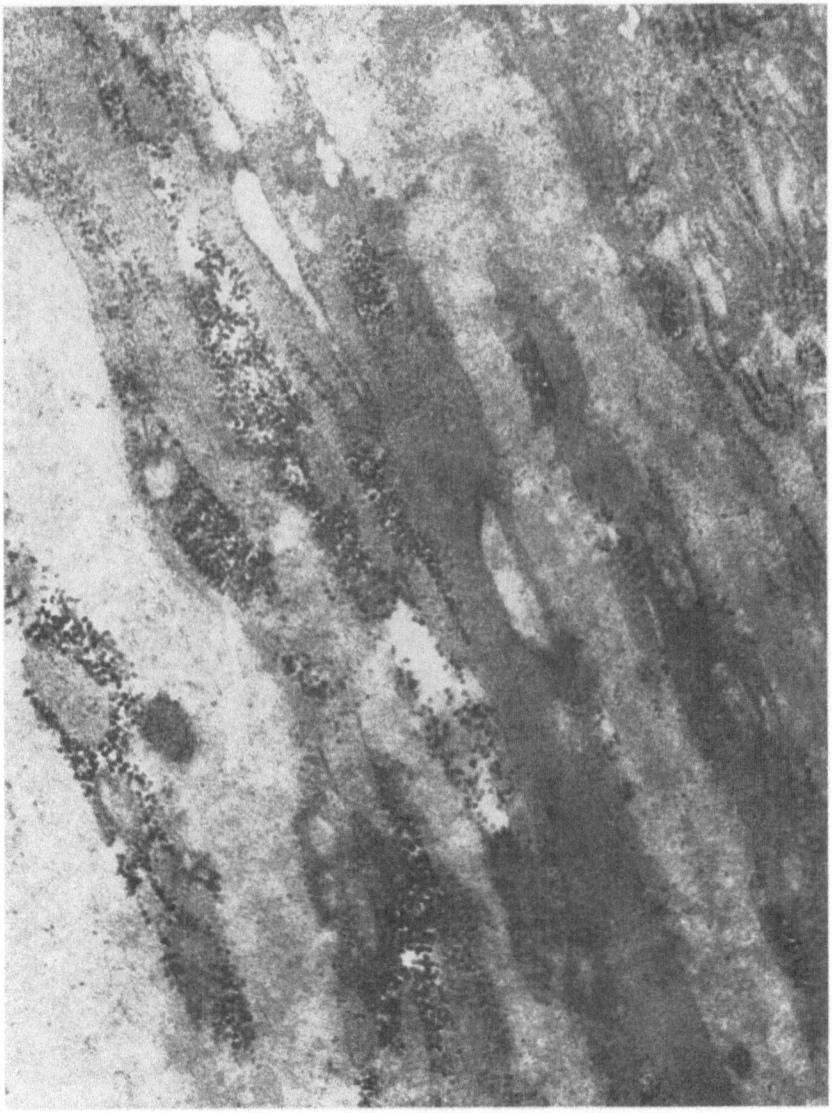

Fig. 23. Development of the ribosomes of the keratocyte twenty-four hours after the incision of the cornea. Transmission electron microscopy (× 8750).

At the electron microscope, we observed a progressive development of the cytoplasmic organelles after the first twenty-four hours. A Golgi's apparatus, some mitochondria and a certain number of dense corpuscles surrounded by a membrane, which were probably lysosomes, were seen (Figs. 23 and 24).

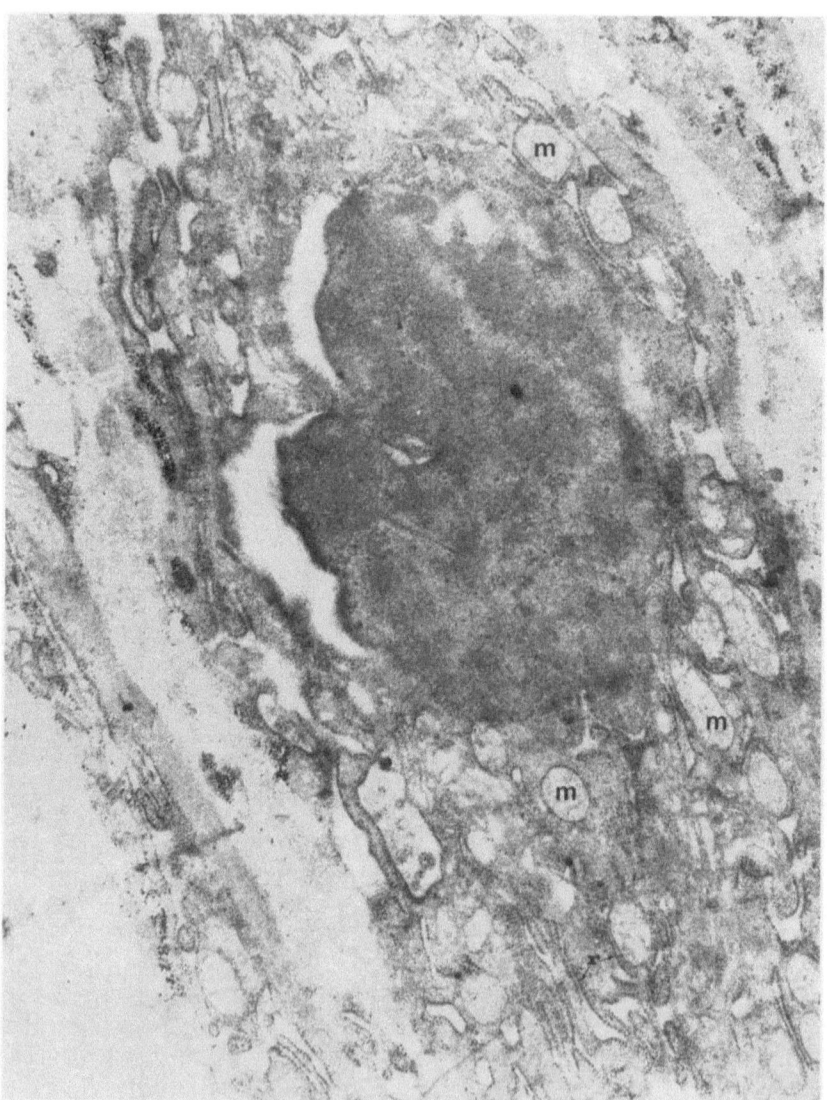

Fig. 24. Keratocyte activated by a corneal wound, forty-eight hours after the incision. Numerous mitochondria (m.) have appeared. Development of the ribosomal endoplasmic reticulum (r.). Transmission electron microscopy (× 6000).

After the fifteenth day, some cells atrophied, but active elements were still found in the third month.

It is interesting to note that the surfaces of the cells were irregular after the first twenty-four hours. After the third day, numerous electron-dense deposits appeared near the cell membrane.

B. Histochemical evolution of the keratocytes in the course of cicatrisation

1) Mucopolysaccharides

The fundamental phenomenon during this period was the appearance of granules of soluble keratosulphate, which can be shown up only by the use of quaternary ammonium salts, such as cetylpyridinium chloride (Table III).

The number of keratosulphate granules increased progressively from the twelfth hour. Already after the first twenty-four hours and until the eleventh day, some clots begun to appear around the cells (Table IV). These extracellular mucopolysaccharides were no longer soluble in water, and they were readily fixed by fixatives that did not contain cetylpyridinium chloride. This fact would indicate that the mucopolysaccharides were free in the granules, but became linked to the proteins as soon as they left the cell. The clots even extended as far as the edge of the wound.

In the cell, the granules occupied the cytoplasm, as well as the pseudopodia. Alongside them, juxtaposed mucopolysaccharides were seen, as if they had just been expelled. These were the deposits, which no longer formed real granules.

From the second day, the keratocytes containing the granules approached nearer and nearer the wound, until they constituted a real cellular mesh-

Table 3. Histochemical characteristics of Kitano's granules (1969).

Toluidine blue in tetraethyl-glycol ether	Toluidine blue in aluminium sulphate	Sky blue	Sudan black	O_5O_4	Nile blue	Pyronin	Fuchsin base
+	+	+	−	−	blue	red	+

Methyl green	Gallocynine	1.2M magnesium chloride	Ribonuclease test
	purple ? RNA	no change in the final Alcian-blue staining	−

−Negative   ++Weakly positive

65

work. By the fifth day, the intercellular spaces were full of a non-hydro-soluble mucopolysaccharidic substance (Table V).

The *metachromatic curves with toluidine blue* were as follows:

1. The metachromasia of the intracellular granules displayed an identi-cal curve after 24, 48 and 72 jours, 4, 5, 8, 11 and 15 days, 1, 2 and 3 months. The maximum of the metachromasia occurred for pH 4.9 and diminished at pH 8.4 and at pH 2.5. The results for the control corneas in tissue culture were the same.

2. On the contrary, for the extracellular material, the maximum meta-chromasia was obtained at pH 6. At lower values of pH, this material be-came almost achromatic, and at higher values of pH (between 7 and 8.4), rather orthochromatic.

After the fifteenth day, the curves became again normal.

Table 4. Histochemistry of corneal wounds twenty-four hours after incision.

Method	Keratocyte cytoplasm	Keratocyte nucleus	Surrounding stroma	Remote stroma
Haematoxylin-eosin-saffron	invisible	normal	oedema	normal
Van Gieson	invisible	normal	yellow	red
Reticulin	–	–	–	++
Metachromatic curve	metachro-matic gra-nules be-tween pH 2 and pH 7.6. Maximum at pH 4.9	normal	slight ortho-chromasia	normal
Colloidal iron	+	–	normal or ++	red
Alcian blue, pH 1	+	–	normal or ++	normal
Alcian blue, pH 2.5	+	--	normal or ++	normal
Alcian blue, pH 6	+	–	normal or ++	normal
Direct Schiff	–	–	–	–
PAS	++	–	normal or ++	+
Feulgen reaction	–	++	some clumps +	–
Acridine orange	red fluo-rescence	green fluores-cence or masked by the red fluo-rescence	some clumps fluorescent green	–
Polarisation microscopy	birefrin-gence –	lacking	lacking	+
Hyaluronidase test	–		–	–
Acid phosphatase	+++	–	– or +	–

–Negative   +Weakly positive   ++Positive   +++Highly positive ⬜ Method inap-plicable

Toward the fifteenth day, the Alcian blue staining of the extracellular structures was negative for 0.1 M concentrations of magnesium chloride.

We found a constant insensitivity to purified bovine testicular hyaluronidase.

At the end of the first month, the metachromasia of the cornea became almost normal, although the values were lower (Table VI). At that time, the keratocytes still contained an abundant cytoplasm with numerous granules.

The stainings of the extracellular mucopolysaccharides were normal.

At the third month, the characteristics of the mucopolysaccharides of the corneal stroma became normal (Table VII).

Table 5. Histochemistry of corneal wounds five days after incision.

Method	Keratocyte cytoplasm	Keratocyte nucleus	Surrounding stroma	Remote stroma
Haematoxylin-eosin-saffron	invisible or pink	basophilia	yellow clumps	increase in keratocytes
Van Gieson	invisible or yellow	normal	yellow or red	increase in keratocytes
Reticulin	apparently cytoplasmic granules	normal	clumps +++	normal
Metachromatic curve	metachromatic granules between pH 2 and pH 7.6 (normal reaction)	normal	deviation toward pH2 to pH 4.9	normal
Colloidal iron	+	normal	++	normal
Alcian blue, pH 1	+	normal	+++	normal
Alcian blue, pH 2.5	+	normal	+++	normal
Alcian blue, pH 6	+	normal	+++	normal
Direct Schiff	normal	normal	−	normal
PAS	+	normal	+++	normal
Oil Red "0"	normal	normal	−	normal
Feulgen reaction	normal	++	normal	normal
Acridine orange	red fluorescence	green fluorescence or masked by red fluorescence	normal	normal
Polarisation microscopy	birefringence-	normal	no birefringence	normal
Hyaluronidase test	normal	normal	normal	normal
Acid phosphatase	+++	normal +	▭	normal

−Negative +Weakly positive ++Positive +++Highly positive ▭ Method inapplicable

67

Table 6. Histochemistry of corneal wounds one month after incision.

Method	Keratocyte cystoplasm	Kerato-cyte nucleus	Surrounding stroma	Remote stroma
Haematoxylin-eosin-saffron	normal	basophilia	normal	number of keratocytes normal or increased
Van Gieson	normal	normal	++	number of keratocytes normal or increased
Reticulin	normal	normal	++	normal
Metachromatic curve	normal	normal	metachromasia persists at lower pH values	normal
Colloidal iron	normal	normal	normal	normal
Alcian blue, pH 1	normal	normal	++	normal
Alcian blue, pH 2.5	normal	normal	++	normal
Alcian blue, pH 6	normal	normal	++	normal
Direct Schiff	–	normal	–	normal
PAS	normal	normal	++	normal
Feulgen reaction	normal	++	normal	normal
Acridine orange	orange fluorescence	normal	normal	normal
Hyaluronidase test	normal	normal	normal	normal
Acid phosphatases	+ or –	normal	normal	normal

–Negative   +Weakly positive   ++Positive

2) *Positive stainings for reticulin*

It is difficult to study reticulin. Nevertheless, it may be said that, from the fifth day, there were positive grumous and fibrillar deposits around the wound (Fig. 25). By the eighth day, these deposits were distinctly fibrillar and by the fifteenth day, the newformed fibres were gradually pushing back the epithelial invagination. At the end of the first month, the wound had an almost normal appearance, although the epithelial invagination was still present. By the third month, there remained a slight epithelial invagination, but the collagen had a normal appearance.

At the *electron microscope*, we observed some electron-dense deposits, located by preference at the periphery, in many cases against the cell membrane.

We can affirm that there existed, for a given number of days after the incision, a parallelism between the positive stainings for reticulin and the quantity of electron-dense deposits observed at the electron microscope; the more positive the stainings in the cytoplasm of the keratocytes, the larger the number of the peripheral electron-dense deposits.

Table 7. Histochemistry of corneal wounds three months after incision.

Method	Keratocyte cytoplasm	Kerato- cyte nucleus	Surrounding stroma	Remote stroma
Haematoxylin-eosin-saffron	normal	normal	normal	normal
Van Gieson	normal	normal	normal	normal
Reticulin	normal	normal	++	normal
Metachromatic curve	normal	normal	normal or persistent metachro- masia at low pH values	normal
Colloidal iron	normal	normal	normal	normal
Alcian blue, pH 1	normal	normal	normal	normal
Alcian blue, pH 2.5	normal	normal	normal	normal
Alcian blue, pH 6	normal	normal	normal	normal
Direct Schiff	−	−	−	−
PAS	normal	normal	++	normal
Oil Red "0"	normal	normal	normal	normal
Feulgen reaction	normal	++	normal	normal
Acridine orange	yellow fluo- rescence	normal	normal	normal
Polarisation microscopy	normal	normal	normal	normal
Hyaluronidase test	normal	normal	normal	normal
Acid phosphatase	normal	normal	normal	normal

−Negative ++Positive

After 4, 5, 8, 11 and 15 days, we made the following observations at the *electron microscope*:

The cytoplasmic organelles were well developed: the mitochondria displayed numerous crests; the reticulo-endoplasmic system was abundant and of the ribosomal type; the Golgi's apparatus might be double and showed a very large number of vesicles.

There were modifications in the cellular membrane: areas of greater density, gaps and blurred edges. In some cases these areas contained very delicate fibrils, such as can be observed in a cell in the course of fibrillogenesis.

Particles of the lysosomal type of about 0.1 μm were also found.

3) *Evolution of the fundamental cellular enzymatic systems*

a) *Acid phosphatases*

In order to obtain indirect, but exclusive, information about the lysosomal activity, we investigated the distribution of the acid phosphatases. In control rabbits with normal corneas, the activity of the acid phosphatases was negative in the keratocytes. On the other hand, the cells of the basal epithelial layer and, in many cases, those of the intermediate epithelial layers, were highly positive.

From the start, a substantial quantity of extracellular enzymes invaded the wound. These enzymes originated most probably in the traumatised epithelium.

After three hours, there was, in addition to the epithelial positivity, an extracellular positivity in the stroma, the keratocytes still remaining negative.

After six hours, the epithelium was still positive, but the keratocytes developed some positive granules. Extracellular acid phosphatase was also found.

After, 9, 12, 15 and 18 hours, the acid phosphatase of the epithelium increased, as it was abundantly found even in the most superficial cells. As to the keratocytes, they accumulated an increasing number of positive granules in their cytoplasm (Fig. 26).

After twenty-four hours, there were intracellular granules. The acid phosphatase was found in the keratocytes remote from the wound.

After 48 and 72 hours, the granules tended to disappear (Fig. 27).

After one month all the layers of the epithelium remained positive. There was no longer any extracellular phosphatase. The keratocytes still contained some positive granules.

After the third month, the distribution of the acid phosphatases in the epithelium became normal again. The keratocytes retained the positive granules. There were no extracellular phosphatases.

These results were identical for both of the methods.

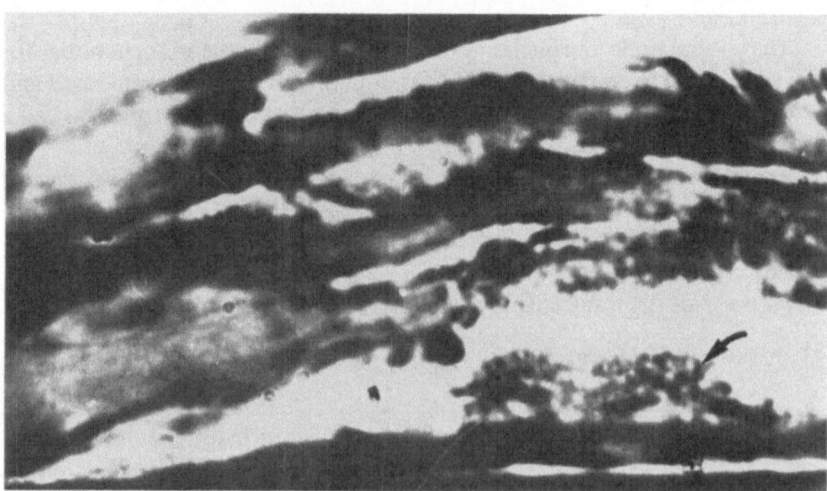

Fig. 25. Transversal section. Keratocyte full of granules positive for reticulin (arrow) on the fifth day after the incision of the cornea. Wilder's staining (x 40 obj.).

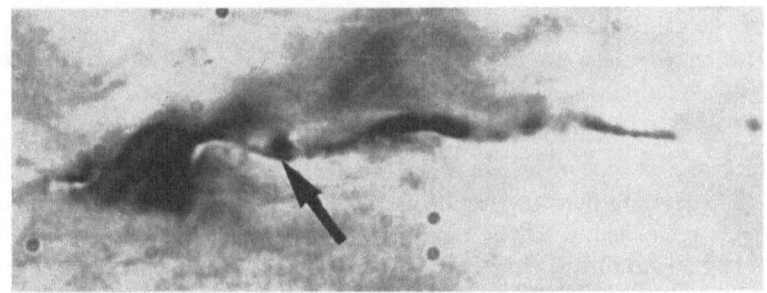

Fig. 26. Granules (arrow) positive for acid phosphatases in the cytoplasm of the keratocytes twenty-four hours after the incision of the cornea. Takeuchi and Tanoue method (x 100 obj.).

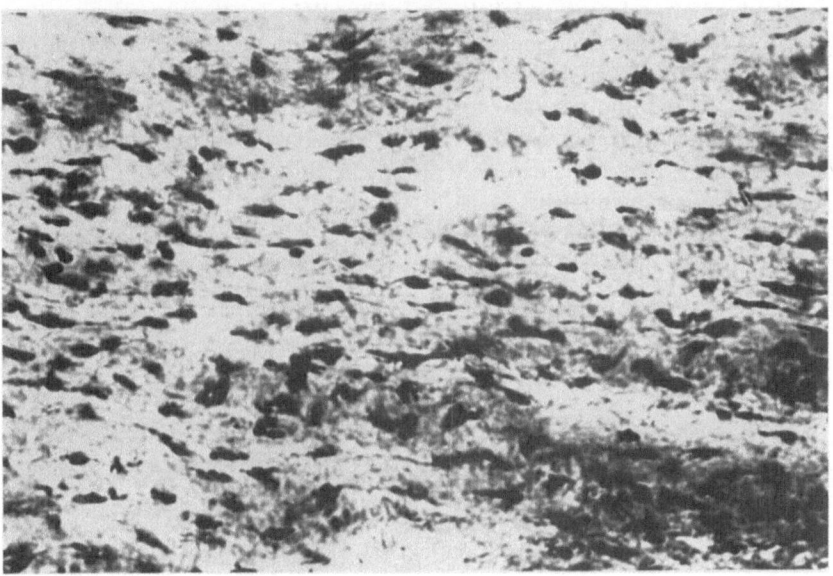

Fig. 27. Numerous keratocytes filled with acid phosphatases four days after the incision. Takeuchi and Tanoue method (x 20 obj.).

b) *β-glucuronidase*

The evolution of the β-glucuronidase was identical with that of the acid phosphatase. This lysosomal enzyme appeared very early, when the keratocyte became an active cell.

c) *Glucose-6-phosphate dehydrogenase*

The histochemical reaction was already positive during the first twelve hours after the activation of the keratocyte.

d) *Lactic dehydrogenase*

This enzyme also was positive during the first hours of the development of active keratocytes.

4) *Phagocytic capacity*

Because the phagocytosis is intimately related with the lysosomal activity, we shall describe here the results obtained. The increase of the acid phosphatases coincided with the development of the phagocytosis, which we tested by means of two vital dyes: neutral red and Trypan blue. The capacity for phagocytosis appeared twelve hours after the incision in all the stromal cells.

5) *Evolution of the nucleic acids.*

As we have already mentioned, we investigated the nucleic acids by the method of Mortelmans and Sebruyns. The RNA in the cytoplasm of the keratocytes increased progressively right from the beginning. After twenty-four hours, there was already a very positive staining. This activity, measured by the red fluorescence of the cytoplasm, attained its maximum at the end of twenty-four hours and became weaker only after one month. By the third month, there remained only an orange fluorescence around the green fluorescence of the nucleus.

The DNA of the nucleus was masked by the intense red fluorescence of the cytoplasm during the first months of the wound healing. On the other hand, the Feulgen nuclear reaction was very intense during the first eight days and diminished thereafter.

We did not notice any negativation of the RNA activity, even after three months. In consequence, the keratocytes remained active.

DISCUSSION AND CONCLUSIONS

The first problem that arises is that of the *origin of the keratocytes* in the corneal wound.

We were able to demonstrate that, when the wound is central and aseptic, the reaction is characterised by, on the one hand, the formation of an epithelial invaginated proliferation and, on the other hand, the activation and the proliferation of the keratocytes.

Wolter (1958) described a cellular reaction consisting of:

1. fixed cells (keratocytes);
2. cells, above all polynuclear cells, originating from the blood;
3. fibroblasts coming from the periphery;
4. perivascular cells in the case of corneal vascularisation;
5. keratocytes passing first through a latency period.

We were able to confirm the conclusions of Weimar (1958), who described a 'lag period' before the cellular proliferation begins. During this latency period, the cell becomes active from the biosynthetic point of view.

Wolter (1958) considered that those cells, originating from the limbus, were lymphocytes, following the Bowman's canals. We know, however, that these canals are only artefacts.

Wolter (1958) described also a transformation of the fixed cells, which lose their star-shape and become fusiform, their nuclei being small and elongated. The fibroblasts of the limbus would be involved only in case of severe stromal traumatism. The silver-carbonate method gives the impression that the keratocytes are not completely differentiated and that they take on a stellar or epithelioid shape. Furthermore, the fibroblasts have a different morphology, even in old corneal scars.

Hanna et al. (1969) found that, after an incision of the cornea, followed immediately by an injection into the anterior chamber of thymidine labelled with tritium, it was the cells surrounding the wound that were the first to become radioactive. That fact argues in favour of a keratocytic origin for most of the cells surrounding the incision.

Robb et al. (1962) described an invasion by leucocytes coming from the precorneal film. That invasion no longer occurs, once the epithelium again covers the wound. For these authors, central corneal wounds contain, apart from the keratocytes, only polynuclear cells, the two types of cells being easily recognisable.

Weimar (1958) investigated in rats the origin of the cells in corneal wounds: 35% of the fibrocytes came from the keratocytes and 65% from the monocytes originating from the limbus. These monocytes would migrate at a speed of 0.29 mm per day. Because the rat's cornea is much smaller, the monocytes can be more easily stimulated by the polypeptides liberated at the level of the wound.

The epithelial cells can remain enclosed within the stroma, but they are never transformed into fibroblasts or keratocytes. This fact was demonstrated by Robb et al. (1964) by radioactive labels applied to the epithelial cells one week before the wound was made.

Kitano (1966) and Goldman (1966) demonstrated the presence of typical keratosulphate granules in the keratocytes. These granules even made it possible to identify the cells.

We found that 80 to 90% of the cells in sterile central corneal wounds consisted of keratocytes from the first hours following the traumatism.

With regard to the *evolution of the mucopolysaccharides*, we observed from the first hours the formation of granules of soluble keratosulphate, which could be demonstrated only after precipitation by quaternary ammonium salts, such as cetylpyridinium chloride (Tables II and III).

Earlier histochemical observations had already shown that the mucopolysaccharides in the keratocytes are formed from the granules described by

Kitano (1966) and Kitano et al. (1966) and confirmed by Payrau et al. (1967). The methods applied before Kitano (1966) produced no fixation of the intracellular mucopolysaccharides, the authors studying only the changes in the underlying stroma. We shall not discuss these changes, our study being limited to the keratocytes.

Kitano et al. (1966) found keratosulphate and chondroitin sulphate in the granules. The keratosulphate disappeared progressively over the first few days. Conversely, in the rabbit we found no chondroitin sulphate A and C, but we did find keratosulphate throughout the duration of the corneal cicatrisation. Payrau et al. (1967) confirmed the presence of chondroitin sulphate A. However, it must not be forgotten that chondroitin sulphate A is sensitive to hyaluronidase. Thus, it should rather be chondroitin sulphate B that was found by these authors. Moreover, as we have already pointed out, the differentiation between keratosulphate and chondroitin sulphate B lies at the limit of the possibilities of the histochemical methods.

We had no opportunity to study the incorporation of S^{35} in Kitano's granules. Dunnington et al. (1958) investigated the fixation of S^{35} at the level of the stroma, but it is possible that S^{35} is fixed first in the granules of the keratocytes, before being found in the stroma. The absence of cetylpyridinium chloride in the fixatives employed prevented any observation of intracellular granules containing S^{35}.

At the electron microscope, the keratocytes 'in situ' previously fixed with cetylpyridinium chloride, displayed electron-dense granules surrounded by a membrane, and having the appearance of lysosomes. That indicates that, morphologically, the mucopolysaccharide granules of the keratocyte should not be very different from lysosomes. They are probably secondary lysosomes.

As we shall see in the next Chapter, the histochemical characteristics of the activated keratocytes are identical with those of the keratocytes in tissue culture.

Unlike the mucopolysaccharides, the reticulin is difficult to demonstrate histochemically in the cytoplasm of the keratocytes 'in situ', because there is no contrast, as a result of the strong positivity of the collagen for Wilder's staining.

We have already pointed out the relative value of Wilder's staining. However, in the case of cicatrisation of corneal wounds, there is a parallel between the positivity of the stainings for reticulin and the presence near the membrane of electron-dense deposits, which appear during the fibrillogenesis of collagen.

Our observations show the early formation of granules of keratosulphate and chondroitin sulphate during the first twenty-four hours. These granules subsequently leave the keratocytes and become extracellular. The formation of mucopolysaccharides precedes that of the collagen precursors (Dunnington, 1957; Dunnington et al., 1958).

Dunnington (1957) and Dunnington et al. (1958) described an increasing deposit of young connective tissue at the level of the wound. That tissue takes on the staining of reticulin and that of picric acid after staining by Van Gieson's method. and this from the fifth day after the incision. We were able to observe the same phenomenon.

We found extracellular collagen from the fifth day onward. It is only slightly stained by PAS, but the positivity of the staining increases during the first days. According to Payrau et al. (1967), the staining is more positive for the mucopolysaccharides associated with the fibrous tissue.

On the other hand, our observations on tissue culture and our histochemical studies, like those of Laurent et al. (1961), suggest the presence of neuraminic acid.

The healing of the cornea is more rapid at the level of the anterior layers (Payrau et al., 1967).

From the ultrastructural point of view, our studies merely confirm the observations of Payrau et al. (1967). In the corneas examined after 4, 5, 8, 11 and 15 days:

1. The keratocyte displays a more extensive cytoplasm. There are numerous very developed mitochondria, multiple Golgi's apparatus and an important ribosomal reticulo-endoplasmic system.

2. At the level of the cellular membrane, there are holes that correspond to the openings of the Golgi's vesicles and extensive areas where the edge of the cell is indistinct; this is visible above all at the level of the pseudopodia.

Fitton-Jackson (1964) described these modifications as a manifestation of fibrillogenesis and did not think that they were real openings.

3. There are juxtacellular formations: (a) normal fibrils, (b) small masses of microfibrils of 80 to 100 Å, (c) diffuse areas of granular material.

Our histochemical study of the *nucleic acids* with acridine orange and the Feulgen reaction, as well as the histochemical studies of Kitano (1966), show activation of the keratocytes throughout the first twenty-four hours after the production of the wound. There is a development of the nucleoli and of the ribosomal endoplasmic reticulum (Payrau et al., 1967). Moreover, the nuclei display a strongly positive Feulgen reaction after the first twenty-four hours.

The *histo-enzymological studies* also indicate an activation of the keratocyte during the healing process of the central corneal wound.

We have not found in the literature any histochemical research relating to the appearance of acid phosphatase and β-glucuronidase during the first hours after the incision. The presence of these enzymes indicates the activation of lysosomes, and it may be supposed that other enzymes of the lysosomal pool appear at the same time. The lysosomal activity persists for at least three months.

We were also able to demonstrate enzymes belonging generally to the mitochondria: glucose-6-phosphate dehydrogenase and lactic dehydrogenase.

Peña Carillo (1963) described an increase of the glucose-6-phosphate dehydrogenase and of the cytochrome oxydase after a homologous or heterologous corneal graft.

According to Weimar et al. (1965), six and twenty-four hours after an incision, the keratocyte develops two enzymatic systems, that of 5-nucleotidase and that of succinodehydrogenase.

The activity of the 5-nucleotidase increases from the first hour until the fourth day and thereafter decreases, until it is no longer found, except in the keratocytes surrounding the wound. On the other hand, the activity of the succino-dehydrogenase continues until the seventh day. Weimar et al. (1966) described the production of an oxidase resistant to formol, sensitive to cyanide and to phenyl hydrazine, but insensitive to azide. This enzymatic system develops in the keratocytes, the epithelial cells and the endothelial cells, at the same time as the 5-nucleotidase system. That system should be specific to the cornea.

By means of nitroblue-tetrazolium Kaufman et al. (1954) found a dehydrogenase in normal corneas and in corneas injured by cold. In the normal corneas, the anterior third was positive, first below the epithelium.

In sutured wounds, Kaufman (1964) found DPN and TPN diaphorases, lactic dehydrogenase, β-glycerophosphate-dehydrogenase and malico-dehydrogenase, accompanied by a decrease of succino-dehydrogenase.

The development of the phagocytosis in the activated keratocytes was demonstrated by Weimar (1958, 1959 and 1962) for two dyes: Trypan blue and neutral red. We were able to confirm these results, but we were also able to demonstrate a parallel between the development of the phagocytic capacity and the evolution of the acid phosphatases. It must not be forgotten that the phagocytosis depends upon the vacuolar system, of which the lysosomes form part. Our results may be summarised chronologically as follows:

At the thirty-sixth hour, the phagocytic capacity decreases in the keratocytes at the edge of the wound.

By the sixtieth hour, the keratocytes at the edge of the wound have lost that capacity. In the more remote keratocytes, it diminishes progressively and is lost toward the hundredth hour.

It is possible that the acid phosphatases, which persist until the third month, are involved only in intracellular activities.

In conclusion:

A. The corneal cicatrisation comprises the following periods:

1. *An epithelial period*, which begins in the first hour. There is a 'massive

discharge' of lysosomal enzymes from the epithelium. Among these enzymes are collagenase and probably the whole of the enzymatic pool capable of acting on the mucopolysaccharides.

2. *A period of enzymatic development*, the 'lag period' of Weimar (1958). During this latency period there is an intense biosynthesis of intracellular elements (mitochondria, etc.). It increases after forty-eight hours, the epithelial action continuing. During this period, the enzymatic systems of the keratocyte develop.

3. *A period of biosynthesis of mucopolysaccharides*, which begins already after twenty-four hours.

4. *A period of division of the keratocytes*, which begins after forty-eight hours.

5. *A period of fibrillogenesis*, characterised by the formation of juxtacellular deposits, which can be demonstrated histochemically from the fifth day.

6. *A period of organisation*, which is very long. By the third month there are still signs of activity in the keratocytes.

7. *A period of involution*, which begins from the fifteenth day on.

All these periods overlap to various extents and can display individual variations.

B. As regards the types of cells, we observed:

1. That when the corneal wound is small and central, the cell population consists almost exclusively of keratocytes (90%), which can be identified by the presence of keratosulphate granules in their cytoplasm.

2. That the keratocytes become active and the cytoplasmic organelles develop.

3. That histochemically RNA and DNA activity becomes apparent, whereas in the normal keratocyte *'in situ'* only DNA activity is found.

4. That the keratocyte displays an early formation of keratosulphate granules, and, later, granules that are positive for reticulin.

5. That the lysosomal system of the keratocytes develops rapidly, as is shown by the positive stainings for acid phosphatases.

6. That the periods of development of all these systems overlap, so that one phase of the cicatrisation may begin, notwithstanding that the preceding one has not yet ended.

77

CHAPTER V

KERATOCYTES IN TISSUE CULTURE

I. INTRODUCTION

In this Chapter we will study the keratocytes in tissue culture from the histochemical and microscopical standpoints. We have found no similar studies in the literature. As a consequence, we can only cite studies in which the culture of the keratocyte was undertaken with different objectives in view.

It is probable Matsui (1928/29) who was the first to cultivate corneal fibroblasts. Although he was trying to obtain cultures of the endothelium, a certain number of fibroblasts developed in the culture.

Thygeson (1939) obtained an important development of fibroblastic cells, after having first obtained a weak growth of epithelial cells. He was also able to obtain fibroblast subcultures.

Histotypical cultures of the cornea have been made for a variety of purposes. The largest developments have been obtained by those who used such cultures in order to *verify the viability of conserved corneal cells* (Draheim et al., 1957; Cockeram et al., 1957; Stocker et al., 1958, 1959 and 1960).

Draheim et al. (1957) compared the viability of corneas frozen at −79°C and after having been immersed in a glycerol bath, with that of corneas which had not undergone any treatment. They obtained positive cultures of the epithelium and keratocytes after forty-eight hours, the best results being obtained with a 10-15% concentration of glycerol. After a month, however, all the cultures were negative.

Cockeram et al. (1957) obtained positive cultures of corneal fibroblasts conserved for three months at −79°C, but only when the freezing was effected gradually. When the freezing was rapid, the viability was zero after $1\frac{1}{2}$ hours of conservation.

Stocker et al. (1958, 1959 and 1960) developed a method for cultivating separately the epithelium, the stroma and the endothelium. The epithelial and endothelial cells developed first and, after a latency period of two or three days, the keratocytes were seen to appear. The keratocytes developed rapidly and smothered the epithelial and endothelial cells. They resisted better freezing. The best method of conserving all the cellular layers of the cornea was congelation at −45°C in a bath of a 20% glycerol solution in physiological saline. In that manner, the cell viability attained sixteen weeks in rabbits.

Harper et al. (1958) made cultures for investigating the influence on the cornea of saline solutions of different types. They made separate cultures of the anterior cornea and of the posterior cornea. In the latter case, they obtained mixed cultures of endothelial cells and keratocytes.

Offret (1955) and Dohlman (1960) made cultures of the cornea in order to study the *development of grafted cells* in cases of corneal transplantation.

Hoof (1948), Sykes et al. (1959), Ehrlich et al. (1961), Halbert et al. (1962) utilised keratocyte cultures for *immunological studies.*

Hoof (1948) cultivated human corneas, as well as those of guinea pigs and chicken embryos. He obtained mixed endothelial and stromal cultures. The cells were shaped like 'medusan heads' and he observed cytoplasmic granulations in the keratocytes. He noted that the keratocytes could develop outside the stroma.

Sykes et al. (1959) implanted pieces of cultivated corneas in rabbits, basing on the theory that precultivated tissues lose a part of their antigenicity. However, they were not real histotypical cultures.

Ehrlich et al. (1961) injected homogenates of the cornea, the lens and the heart in ducks. The activity of the anti-sera was controlled in tissue culture (in 'lying drops') and observed between two cover-slips. The keratocytes were impaired by all sera. It was the serum prepared from the corneal epithelium that caused most damage to the cultivated cells.

Soltz et al. (1961) implanted in the same flask fragments of corneas of different origins. When the growth areas became contiguous, there was an inhibition of the development in the case of two human corneas from different subjects. When one of the implants was human and the other from a mouse, it was the human fragment that was inhibited.

Basu et al. (1960) and Sarkar et al. (1962), using rabbits, made cultures of keratocytes in order to study the *caryograms* and the sexual chromatin. They made corneal transplantations between donors and receivers of different sexes. They concluded that the donors' cells persist for about three months in the receiver, being progressively replaced by the keratocytes of the latter.

Sarkar et al. (1962) also studied the caryotypes of the cultivated rabbit keratocytes. They concluded that:

1. The keratocytes and the endothelial cells conserve their own morphology after several subcultures.

2. The number of keratocyte chromosomes is 44, including the XX and XY chromosomes.

3. The chromosomes may be grouped according to their dimensions, but they cannot be individualised.

4. The Y chromosome of the male rabbit is similar to the two smallest autosomes.

5. The chromosomes 18 and 19 are telocentric and the most easily individualisable.

Much research has been done on keratocyte cultures in the field of *virology*, but infections do not concern us in the present study.

Lucas (1965) made both histotypical and organotypical cultures of all the ocular tissues.

Fowle et al. (1955) and François et al. (1973 and 1974) studied the keratocytes in tissue culture both cytochemically and microscopically. We shall report in greater detail on the results in this chapter.

While studying the healing of corneal wounds, Wolter (1958) demonstrated a dedifferentiation of keratocytes in fibroblasts. Was that dedifferentiation purely morphological or did it involve also the biosynthesis of the cell elements?

Kitano (1966 and 1969) studied histochemically the keratosulphate granules of the activated keratocytes in corneal wounds. But what are the characteristics of the keratocytes activated by tissue culture?

After the biosynthesis of reticulin, are the granules containing it, the same as those which store the mucopolysaccharides?

It is to reply to these questions and in order to investigate their histochemical properties and their biosynthesis capacity that we cultivated keratocytes in pure tissue culture.

II. PERSONAL OBSERVATIONS

A. Examination of the primary cultures
in vivo during growth

Already at the end of forty-eight hours, numerous keratocytes were seen, proliferating between the lamellae of the cornea. At the end of seventy-two hours, the cells proliferated at the edge of the specimen (Fig. 28). On the fourth day, the proliferation continued and occurred on two or three planes. The keratocytes tended to form a meshwork, which developed still further on the fifth and sixth days, the meshes becoming ever more tightly pressed together, so that, toward the seventh day, a veritable carpet of cells was obtained.

During this period of growth, it was observed that the cytoplasm was granulated and that the nuclei were very active, containing more than three nucleoli.

Microcinematographical studies showed that the keratocytes migrated rather slowly in the specimen and much more rapidly on the wall of the culture flask. In the first case, the keratocyte covered 1 μm in 2.15 minutes; in the second case, 1 μm in 1.40 minutes.

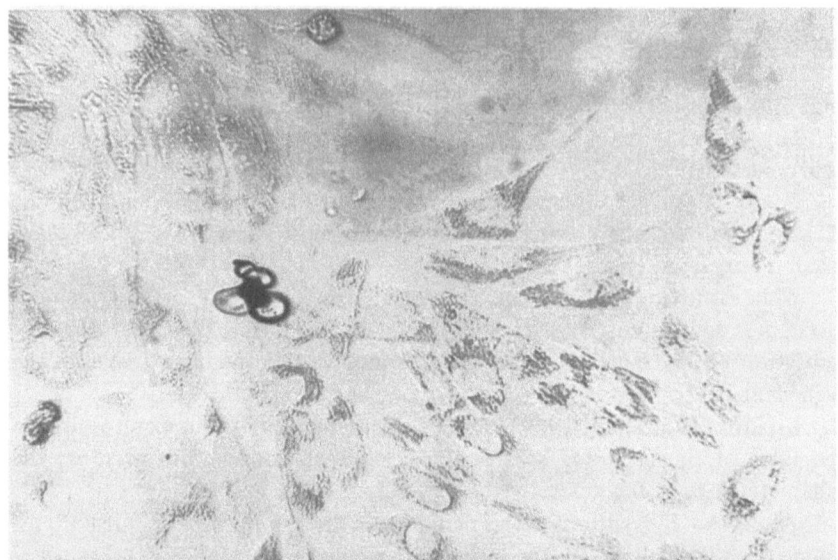

Fig. 28. Primoculture of keratocytes. Development of intracytoplasmic granules (grey). Phase-contrast microscopy (x 20 obj.).

B. *Examination of the subcultures*
in vivo during growth

If the cells in the culture flask were examined immediately after trypsinisation, it was seen that they rapidly took on a fibroblastic appearance. The cytoplasm displayed numerous granules, either close to the two poles of the nucleus or around the nucleus (Figs. 29 and 30). By microcinematography, one could see the granules moving rapidly in all directions, carried by the cytoplasmic currents.

In the subcultures, the cellular proliferation was very rapid. Forty-eight to seventy-two hours after the first trypsinisation, it became necessary to retrypsinise, because the cells formed a carpet, which begun to detach at the borders. After a second or a third trypsinisation, the cells continued to divide, and their cytoplasm still contained a large number of granules.

C. *Examination at the phase-contrast microscope of*
living monolayers, mounted in Ringer's solution

Keratocytes in monolayers had the appearance of fibroblasts with long pseudopodia. When the cells were in different planes, these tentacles could pass underneath other cellular bodies, but there existed also real intercellular cytoplasmic bridges.

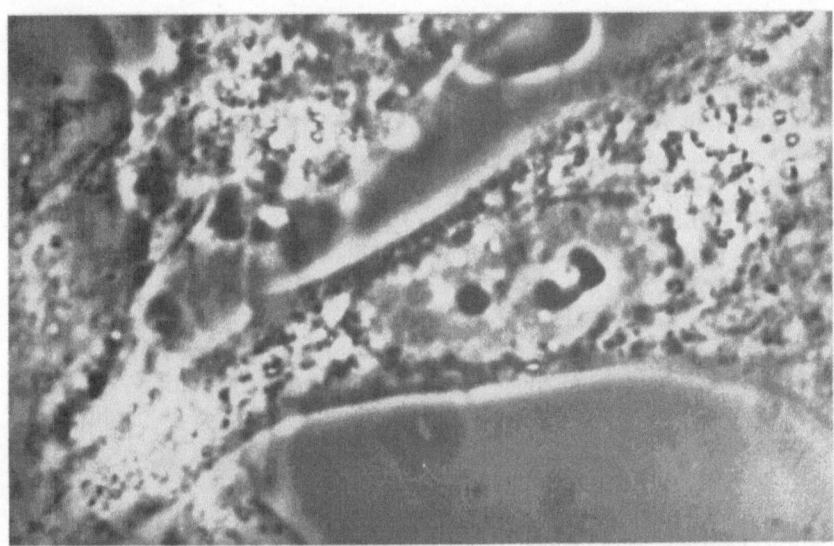

Fig. 29. Monolayer of keratocytes in culturc. Intracytoplasmic granules (black) and vacuoles (white). Nucleus with two nucleoli. Phase-contrast microscopy (× 100 obj.).

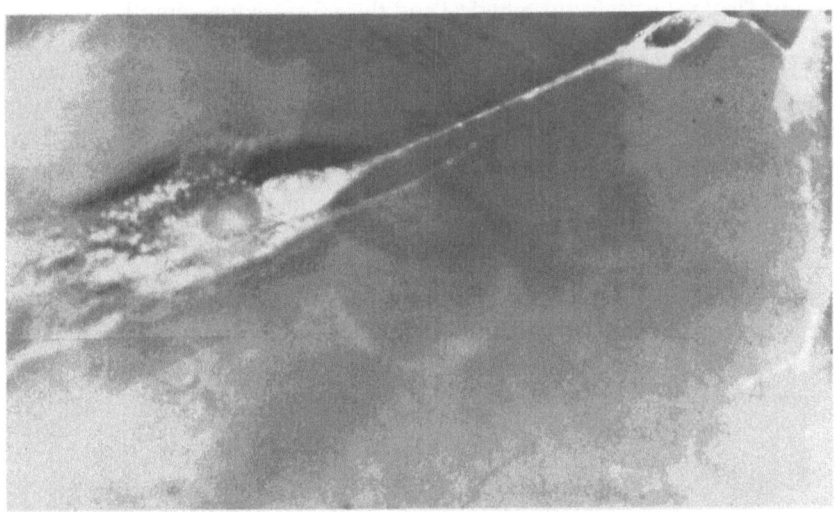

Fig. 30. Living normal keratocyte in tissue culture. Oval formation in one pole of the cell. This formation contains vacuoles and granules. Relief phase-contrast microscopy (× 40 obj.).

The shapes of the keratocytes were often stellar or fusiform. Cytoplasmic extensions, taking on the appearance of a transparent veil, were arranged like a fan around the cellular body. In some cases these fine extensions travelled a long distance before attaching themselves to the glass wall.

The nuclei were oval and contained from one to five nucleoli.

The dimensions of the keratocytes varied depending upon the shape of the cells, which were always flattened. The star-shaped cells had cellular bodies measuring about 30 μm and triangular extensions which also measured from 30 to 40 μm. The fine extensions might be as long as 100 μm. The nuclei measured 8x 13 μm.

In many cases the surface of the cells was irregular, displaying fine folds.

The keratocytes were highly mobile; amoeboid and undulatory movements were observed, particularly visible during microcinematographical observation.

The cytoplasm of the keratocytes contained a very large number of elements (Figs. 29 and 30). First of all, there were *granules*. Although, in some cells, they were arranged at the two poles of the nucleus, sometimes by adhering to the nuclear membrane; in others they occupied the whole extent of the cytoplasm as far as inside the pseudopodia. At the instant of the secretion of the granule contents, the granules coalesced to form a very characteristic mass having the dimensions of the nucleus. Some granules remained disseminated in the cytoplasm.

The granules measured between 0.2 and 0.5 μm. They might be isolated, but more commonly, they constituted small groups measuring between 1 and 3 μm. They were perfectly spherical and their surface was smooth.

Then there were white *vacuoles*, which were very numerous. They were arranged between the granules and were in many cases perinuclear. Their shapes and dimensions were various and irregular. Their longest axes measured between 0.5 and 4 μm.

The bond between the cell cytoplasm and the wall of the flask was in some cases strong, measuring a few microns in thickness, in other cases nevertheless very slight.

The nuclei appeared very active. Their chromatin was finely granulated. Each contained from one to five irregular, rounded nucleoli, measuring between 1 and 2 μm. The nuclear membrane was very fine.

The *intercellular bridges* were very thin and contained granules. Their diameters ranged from 0.2 to 0.3 μm, their lengths being variable.

III. HISTOCHEMICAL STUDY (Table VIII)

The results of our histochemical studies are summarised in Table VIII (Figs. 31 and 32).

The granules containing reticulin were different from those containing

Table 8. Normal keratocytes in tissue culture.

Histochemical staining	Soluble granules	Insoluble granules	Vacuoles	Cytoplasmic matrix	Nucleus	Nucleoli
PAS	++	++	–	+ in places	–	–
Alcian blue, pH 1	+	+	–	–		
Alcian blue, pH 2.5	+	+	–	–		
Colloidal iron	+	+	–	–		
Metachromatic curve for toluidine blue	+ metachromasia between pH 2 and pH 7.2	+ between pH 5 and pH 7.5	achromasia	+ metachromasia between pH 5 and pH 7.5	orthochromasia	orthochromasia
Reticulin according to Wilder	++ for some	++ for some	–	+		
Van Gieson	–	–	–	–		
Haematoxylin-eosin	The cytoplasm shows a uniform eosinophilia				+ basophilia	+ basophilia
Oil Red "0"	–	–	+	–		
Feulgen nuclear reaction	–	–	–	–	–	+
Acridine orange	Intense and persistent red fluorescence in all the cytoplasm with visualisation of the ergastoplasm				green fluorescence	red or orange fluorescence
Ribonuclease				+	–	+
Hyaluronidase test controlled with pH 6.2 toluidine blue	–	–				
Activity of the acid phosphatases	Presence of numerous positive cytoplasmic granules					

– Negative   + Weakly positive   ++ Positive   ☐ Method inapplicable

85

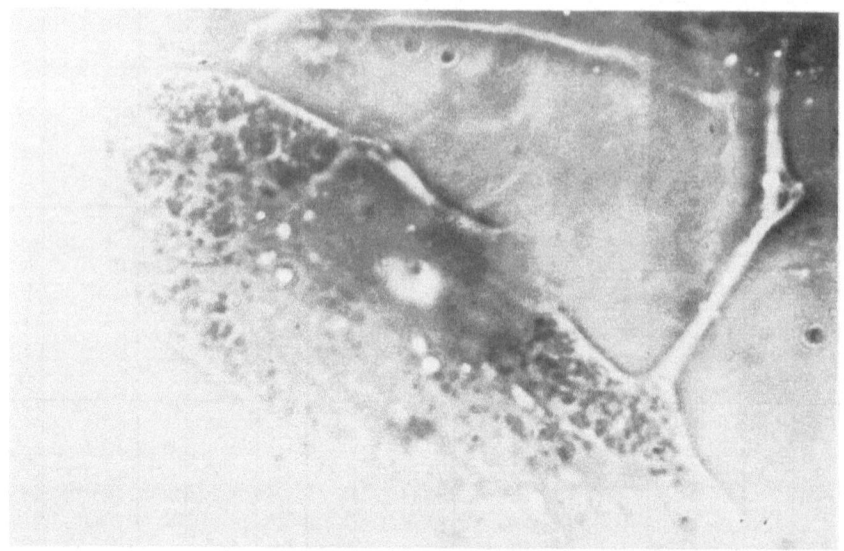

Fig. 31. Normal keratocyte in tissue culture. Numerous mucopolysaccharide granules (black). PAS staining. Phase-contrast microscopy (x 1000 obj.).

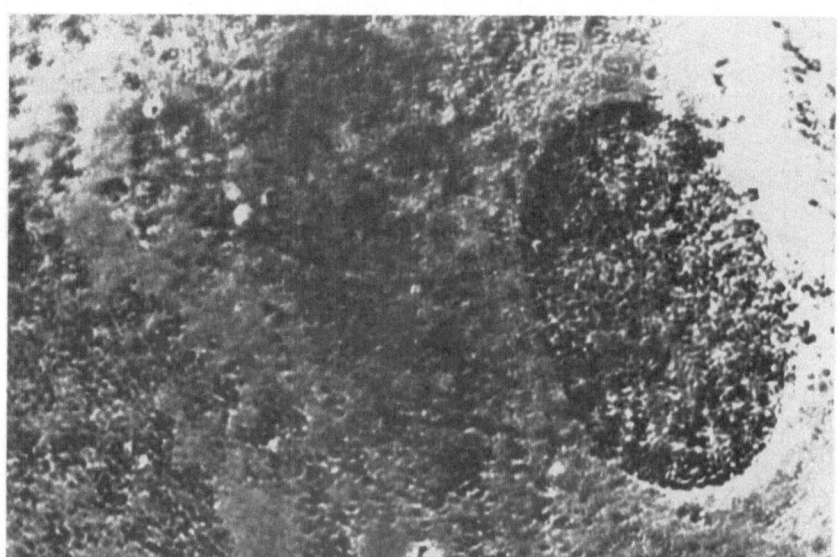

Fig. 32. Normal keratocyte in tissue culture. Granules containing reticulin. Wilder's reticulin method. Phase-contrast microscopy (x 1000 obj).

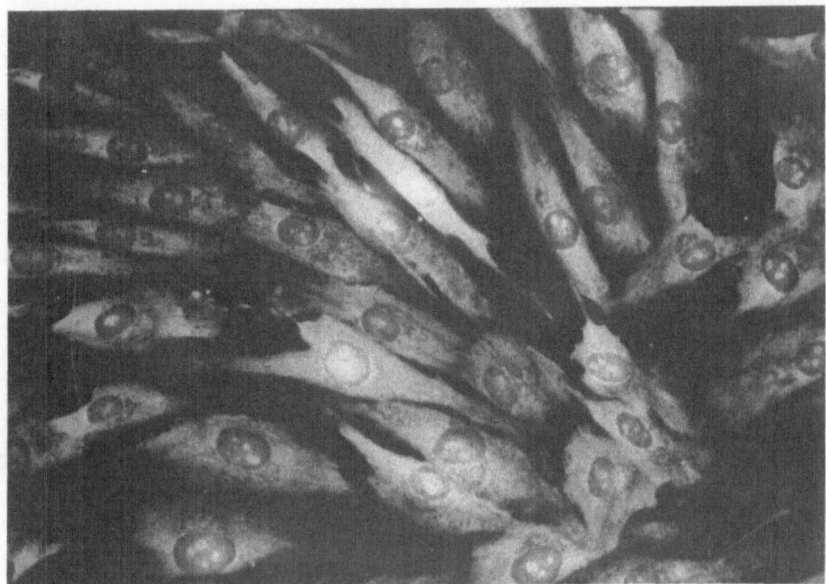

Fig. 33. Normal keratocyte in tissue culture. The orange-red fluorescence of the cyto-plasm and the nucleoli indicates RNA. The DNA shows a green fluorescence. Fluores-cence microscopy (x 20 obj.).

mucopolysaccharides. The former were found, indeed, for preference close to the cell surface, whereas the latter were more commonly found near the nucleus. The PAS-positive part of the cytoplasmic matrix corresponded eith-er to mucopolysaccharides in solution, or to neuraminic acid, which is abun-dant in the corneal stroma. The reticulin of the cytoplasmic matrix was represented by particles that were at the limit of visibility at the clear-field microscope, but clearly visible at the dark-field microscope.

The vacuoles contained lipids.

The staining by acridine orange showed high biosynthesis activity, at the level of the nucleoli as well as at that of the cytoplasm, whose RNA-positive ergastoplasm was highly developed (Fig. 33).

A fundamental characteristic of the keratocytes in tissue culture was the presence of keratosulphate in the soluble granules, which could be fixed only with formol or cetylpyridinium chloride.

Depending upon the fixative used, it was possible to find:

1. Granules containing mucopolysaccharides and above all keratosulphate, which is characteristic of the cornea. These granules were soluble, but could be fixed.

2. Insoluble granules, positive to PAS and colloidal iron, which contained glycoproteins and/or neuraminic acid.

3. Insoluble granules containing reticulin.

87

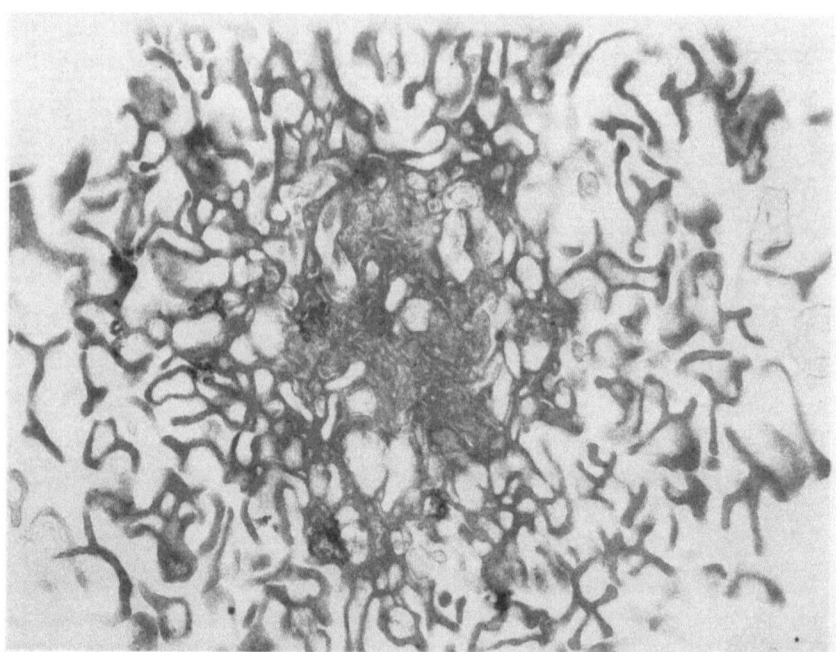

Fig. 34. Transversal section of a cultivated keratocyte in suspension. There are numerous cytoplasmic extensions (pseudopodia). Transmission electron microscopy (x 3000).

In the mitochondria, stainings positive for glucose-6-phosphate dehydrogenase and lacto-dehydrogenase were observed.

In the lysosomes, the study of which *'in vitro'* will be described later, stainings positive for acid phosphatase and β-glucuronidase could be observed.

IV. TRANSMISSION ELECTRON MICROSCOPY

When the keratocytes in tissue culture were observed at the transmission electron microscope, little difference from other cultivated fibroblasts was evident. We studied cells spread on a plastics surface and cells in suspension. In the latter case, they took on the appearance of medusae with numerous pseudopodia arranged radially (Fig. 34).

At the level of the *cytoplasm* could be seen:

1. Numerous granulations of velvety appearance and variable electron density. They were surrounded by a membrane (Fig. 35).
2. Mitochondria with numerous transversal crests.
3. A highly developed Golgi's apparatus containing numerous flattened cisterns and numerous vacuoles of various sizes, and

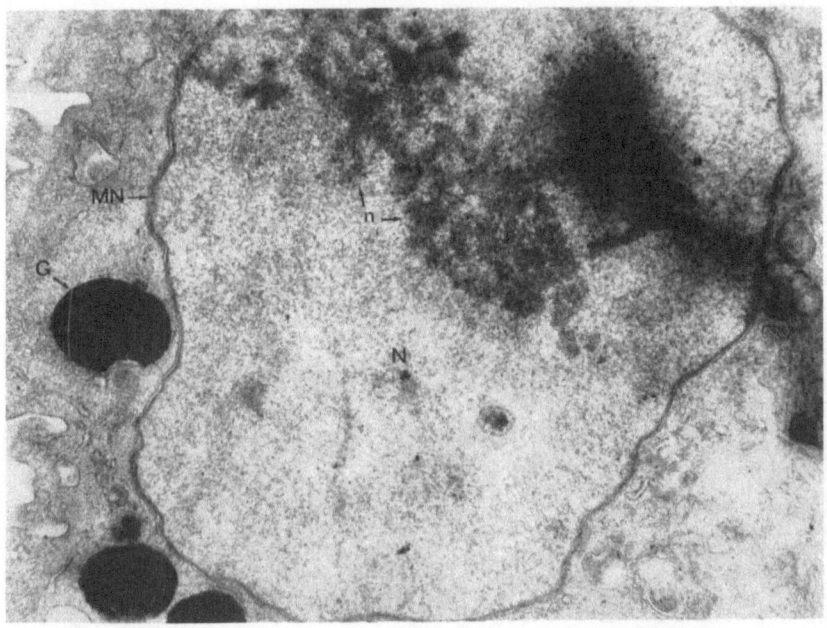

Fig. 35. Keratocyte in tissue culture. (N) nucleus containing nucleolar material. (G) electron-dense granules. Transmission electron microscopy (x 13 740).

4.   A finely granular cytoplasmic matrix.

At the level of the *nucleus* could be seen (Fig. 35):

1.   Typical nucleoli displaying nucleolonemes, whose granular and filamentary parts were not separated (unseggregated type), and

2.   A dense and grouped chromatin, located in many cases against the nuclear membrane.

V.   SCANNING ELECTRON MICROSCOPY

The specimen displayed anfractuous borders at the places where the keratocytes emerged. The latter became flattened on the glass slide (Fig. 36).

The cytoplasm was stretched by the tonofibrils. It displayed numerous pseudopodia both of the first order, emerging from the cell body, and of the second order, emerging from the first-order pseudopodia. The bonding to the glass slide was effected by very fine cytoplasmic ties.

The nucleus was highly developed and displayed prominent nucleoli of spherical shape (Fig. 36).

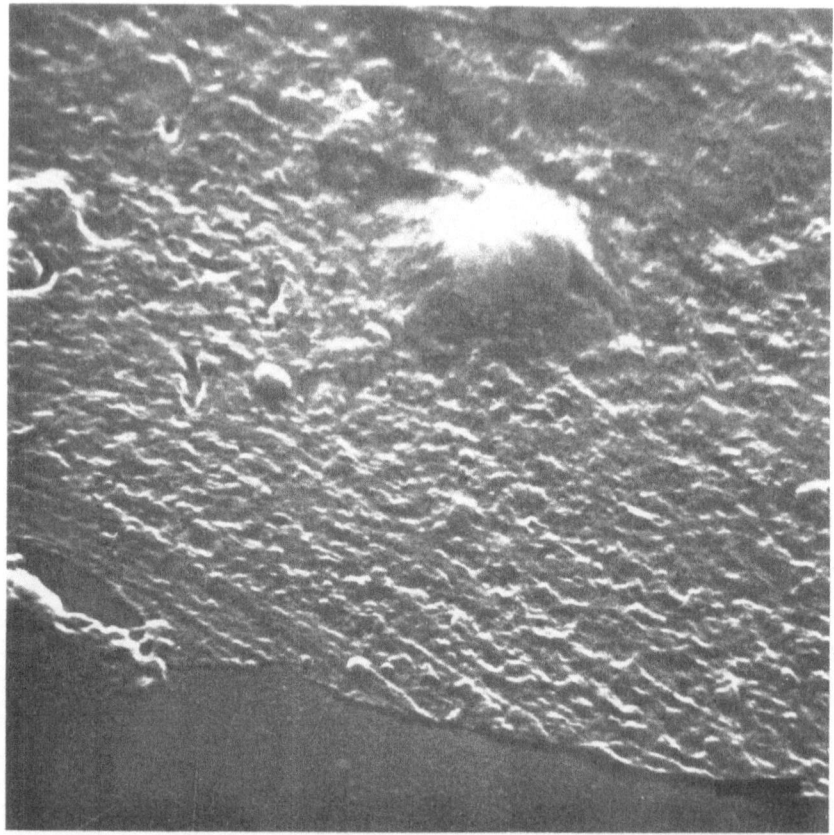

Fig. 36. Keratocyte in tissue culture. The cytoplasm shows numerous tonofibrils. The nucleolus is prominent. Scanning electron microscopy (x 3724).

VI. DISCUSSION AND CONCLUSIONS

The culture of keratocytes rendered it possible to study the histochemical characteristics of the various elements of the active cells, which is very difficult to achieve with cells *in situ* in the corneal stroma.

The development of keratocytes in culture occurs in successive phases, similar to those that are observed in the cicatrisation of corneal wounds (Weimar, 1958; Kitano, 1969).

Our studies show that the characteristics of keratocytes in culture are the following:

1. The presence of granules containing keratosulphate. These soluble granules correspond exactly to the intra- and extra-cellular granules described by Kitano (1966, 1969) in the healing of corneal wounds.

2. The presence of vacuoles containing lipids. These might be proteolipids,

that is to say, an association of proteins and lipids. Their histochemical characteristics are, however, those of lipids.

The dedifferentiation of the keratocytes into fibroblasts, described by Wolter (1958), is only a morphological change, characterised by the formation of pseudopodia, when the cells have the possibility to spread on a surface. In the culture flasks, all the keratocytes have a fibroblastic appearance, although they display the histochemical characteristics of keratocytes.

The tendency of the keratocytes to form syncytia is demonstrated in tissue culture. Indeed, numerous intercytoplasmic bridges, in some cases containing granules, are observed.

The high RNA activity shows that the stimulated keratocytes can resume a very substantial biosynthetic activity without in any way being dedifferentiated.

The vacuoles containing lipids or proteolipids have also been found in hyalocytes (François et al., 1972d). In addition, keratocytes in culture resemble much more hyalocytes in culture than fibroblasts, the three kinds of cells deriving, however, from the same blastocytes.

The polarity of the granules and the vacuoles, accumulated in the keratocytes after biosynthesis, show that these active cells behave like real glandular cells. In tissue culture, indeed, in some but not all cases, the formation of a secretion pole is seen.

The positivity for acid phosphatases and β-glucuronidase shows that the keratocytes are capable of developing a lysosomal system, indispensable for the catabolic activities.

We can conclude that two types of granules are present:
1. Those that contain mucopolysaccharides. They are rather perinuclear, but are also found in the cytoplasmic extensions. They are fixed by cetylpyridinium chloride. The PAS positivity in the matrix is probably due to the presence of neuraminic acid, which could already been isolated biochemically.
2. The insoluble granules, which are located at the periphery of the cytoplasm. They are PAS negative, but take on the dyes for reticulin and in some cases, the collagen dyes (Van Gieson).

We found that the products of the collagen biosynthesis are stored in granules which differ from the granules containing mucopolysaccharides. This fact is explained, since the reticulin (precursor of the collagen) is synthesised by the ribosomes, whereas the mucopolysaccharides are synthesised by the Golgi's apparatus.

The definitive collagen of the cornea is produced as a result of an orderly precipitation of precollagen substances in the presence of mucopolysaccharides and other materials of the ground substance.

The presence of G-6-P dehydrogenase and of lactic-dehydrogenase indicates that the glucose can be metabolised aerobically, as well as anaerobically, what confirms the physiological findings.

The transmission electron microscope shows granulations surrounded by membranes. These granulations correspond either to mucopolysaccharide granules or to lysosomes, or, again, to the fusion of both (secondary lysosomes).

The development of the Golgi's apparatus is explained, on the one hand, by the magnitude of the vacuolar system and, on the other hand, by the large-scale production of mucopolysaccharides.

The scanning electron microscope merely confirms the observations made at the phase-contrast microscope.

PART TWO

PATHOLOGIC KERATOCYTES

(MACULAR DYSTROPHY OF THE CORNEA)

CHAPTER VI

I. DEFINITION OF MACULAR DYSTROPHY OF THE CORNEA

Macular dystrophy of the cornea is a primary heredo-familial thesauris-mosis of the keratocytes, accompanied by an accumulation of sulphated mucopolysaccharides. During the evolution of the disease, other layers of the cornea can also be involved.

II. CLINICAL CHARACTERISTICS (Fig. 37)

The affection was described by Groenouw (1890) and Fehr (1904). It is sometimes termed Groenouw's dystrophy type II, type I being the granular dystrophy of the cornea.

The onset of the disease occurs during the first decade of life, between five and nine years (Duke-Elder, 1965; François, 1966).

The biomicroscope shows, during the early years, a diffuse opacity of the superficial and central layers of the cornea, the surface of which be-comes irregular and dull. During the second decade of life, more differ-entiated and denser maculae are seen in the diffuse opacity. At the same time, the lesions spread in depth and toward the periphery. Condensations underneath the epithelium give an even more irregular appearance to the epithelial surface. After the age of about thirty years, the whole thickness of the stroma is affected by a process of opacification and oedema.

The posterior limiting membrane has in some cases the appearance of a cornea guttata (John, 1928; Bücklers, 1938; Van Canneyt et al., 1948; Dededimos, 1950). This endothelial change is compensated, because the stroma displays no diffuse oedema by imbibition. The thickness of the cornea, moreover, remains more or less normal (0.42 mm, according to Malbran et al., 1973).

Although Klintworth et al. (1964), Duke-Elder (1965), Morgan (1966), François (1966), Teng (1966), Malbran (1972), Malbran et al. (1978) found mucopolysaccharides in the endothelium, that can be only a secondary phenomenon. Indeed:

a) The appearance of a cornea guttata is late. It develops only when the deep layers of the stroma are affected.

b) It has not been demonstrated that the corneal endothelium can produce keratosulphate.

95

In the end stage, there are irregularities in the thickness of the cornea, a diminution of the corneal sensitivity, crises of photophobia and irritation as well as recurrent erosions (Duke Elder, 1965).

Between thirty and forty years of age, the patients become practically blind, although in certain cases the vision is compromised only much later (Franceschetti et al., 1950).

The most important differential diagnosis has to be made with granular dystrophy of the cornea. The fundamental difference is that, during the evolution, the macular dystrophy expands peripherically as far as the limbus, and in depth as far as the Descemet's membrane. Furthermore, in granular dystrophy, the spaces between the opacities are clear.

III. HEREDITY

Macular dystrophy is indeed transmitted as a autosomal recessive trait (François, 1966) (Fig. 38):

1. Consanguinity of the parents is frequent.
2. Only brothers and sisters are affected, the disease not being found in either the ascendants or the descendants.
3. About 25% of the sibs are affected.

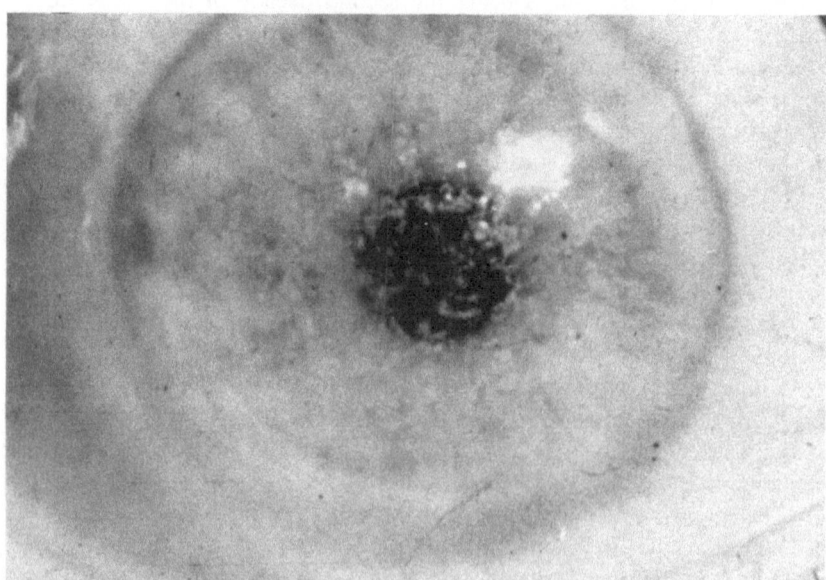

Fig. 37. Clinical aspect of macular dystrophy of the cornea.

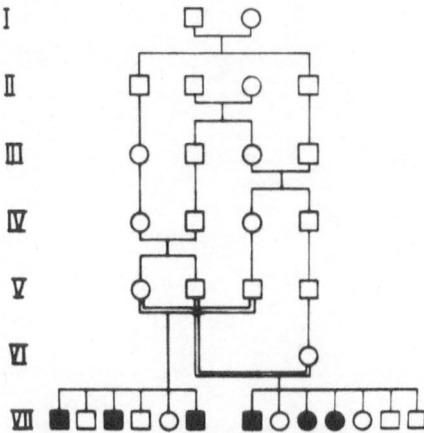

Fig. 38. Macular dystrophy of the cornea. Autosomal recessive inheritance with consanguinity of the parents (after Blum, 1945).

While macular dystrophy of the cornea is autosomal recessive, granular dystrophy is autosomal dominant and this fact makes also possible a differential diagnosis.

CONCLUSIONS

Macular dystrophy of the cornea is a disorder which evolves slowly and progressively. It rapidly impairs the vision. It is characterised by the appearance of irregular opacities in the anterior and central regions of the cornea, thereafter involving the periphery as well as the deepest corneal layers. It has an autosomal recessive inheritance.

CHAPTER VII

MICROSCOPICAL AND HISTOCHEMICAL STUDY
OF MACULAR DYSTROPHY OF THE CORNEA

In this Chapter, we shall restrict ourselves to the study of the changes in the stroma and, more particularly, in the keratocytes. The changes of the epithelium and of the posterior limiting membranes will be described separately.

PERSONAL OBSERVATIONS

A. *Phase-contrast microscopy of fresh sections and of sections fixed before and after dehydration*

Both in frozen sections and in pieces fixed by fixatives containing or not cetylpyridinium chloride, the appearance was similar.

Bowman's membrane was fibrillar or lacking over wide areas. The superficial stroma displayed mostly very extensive pathological areas. Of irregular shapes, they could measure up to 2 mm. They contained a granular material, as well as zones of homogeneous aspect and hyalinised appearance. At the edges of the lesion, there were fringed collagenous lamellae. These areas could be followed on seriated sections. They corresponded without doubt to the dense opacities seen at the biomicroscope. The absence of Bowman's membrane and the irregularity of the affected zones explained the irregularities of the corneal surface, which can be observed clinically. The stroma surrounding these areas was oedematous, as the collagen fibres of the lamellae were dissociated. In the deeper layers of the stroma, interlamellar deposits and pathological keratocytes were observed.

In transverse sections, the interlamellar deposits had a flattened shape, which followed the interlamellar space. They measured from 10 to 50 μm. They consisted of a granular material, each granule measuring approximately 1 μm, as could be deducted from the densitometric measurements. The study of seriated sections demonstrated that they were interlamellar deposits and not keratocytes sectioned parasagitally alongside the nucleus. The stroma immediately above and below had in some cases a normal appearance, and in other cases an oedematous appearance.

On flat sections, the pathologic areas had irregular shapes. They could join up by means of branches which were also irregular.

The keratocytes were of two types:

Table 9. Histochemistry of macular dystrophy of the cornea.

Method	Large subepithelial deposits	Interfascicular deposits	Karatocyte granules	Excrescences of the Descemet's membrane	Granules of endothelial cells
Saffron	unstained	unstained	unstained	reddish yellow	unstained
Van Giesson solution with trinitrophenol and acid fuchsin	unstained	unstained	unstained	red	unstained
Trichrome according to Gomori	unstained	unstained	unstained	reddish	unstained
Reticulin according to Wilder	–	–	–	–	–
Colloidal iron	+	+	+	–	+
Alcian blue, pH 1	+	+	+	–	+
Alcian blue, pH 2.5	+ or –	+ or –	–	–	+ or –
Metachromatic curve	metachromasia at all pH values	metachromasia at all pH values		metachromasia between pH 4 and pH 6.8	metachromasia at all pH values
Direct Schiff	negative	negative		–	–
PAS	+	+	+	–	–
Saunder's method	+ for keratosulphate			–	+ for keratosulphate
Neutralisation of the Alcian blue by magnesium-chloride	Alcian blue + up to a magnesium-chloride concentration of 1 to 1.3 M	Alcian blue + up to a magnesium-chloride concentration of 1 to 1.3 M			Alcian blue + up to a magnesium-chloride concentration of 1 to 1.3 M
Action of hyaluronidase	–	–	–	–	–

–Negative +Weakly positive ▢ Method inapplicable

Table 10. Histochemistry of macular dystrophy of the cornea.
Second Part

Method	Large subepithelial deposits	Interfascicular deposits	Keratocyte granules	Excrescences of the Descemet's membrane	Granules of endothelial cells
Toluidine blue in aluminium sulphate	++	++	++	–	++
Nile blue	+	+	+	–	+
Pyronine	+	+	+	–	+
Mortelmans and Sebruyns' method for the nucleic acids	There is no DNA or RNA activity				
Oil Red "0", Sudan black and Sudan III	–	–	–	–	–
Acid phosphatases	+	++	++	++	++
Takeuchi and Tanoue Method	+	++	++	++	++
Polarisation microscopy	no birefringence	"spherite" configuration	"spherite" configuration	slight + birefringence	"spherite" configuration
Dark-field microscopy	some refringent dots	Refringent dots	Refringent dots	Optical vacuity	Refringent dots
Phase-contrast microscopy	Homogeneous	clear granules	clear granules	Reddish	clear granules

–Negative +Weakly positive ++Positive

a. *Some of them had a nucleus of normal appearance*, but a cytoplasm full of granules similar to those of the interlamellar deposits. In some cases these granules gave them a globular appearance, but more often an oval shape. The volume of these keratocytes was several times greater than that of normal cells; they measured from 15 to 40 μm.

b. *Other keratocytes had picnotic nuclei.* In these cases, the number of granules was much greater. Their cytoplasm was most often globular, pressing back the neighbouring structures. The nucleus was reduced to a small dense mass of irregular shape.

On flat sections, these keratocytes had shapes and arrangements similar to those of the interlamellar deposits. Their granular material was, moreover, identical with that of the interlamellar deposits. The morphological appearance seemed to indicate that these interlamellar deposits were, in fact, merely degenerated keratocytes that had lost their nuclei.

B. Optical microscopy of histochemically stained sections (Tables IX and X)

When sections were stained, either frozen sections or sections fixed with formol buffered with pH 7.2 phosphate, with or without cetylpyridinium chloride or sections fixed with glutaraldehyde buffered with pH 7.2 cacodilate, the following observations might be made:

1. *Sections stained with haematoxylin-eosin-saffron.* The nuclei were stained blue. Numerous nuclei were picnotic, showing a concentrated chromatin; others had a more normal appearance, displaying a finely granulated chromatin.

The superficial deposits could show a slight eosinophilia at the level of the homogeneous areas.

The granulations that filled the cytoplasm of the keratocytes or the interlamellar deposits were negative for haematoxylin, eosin and saffron. The last-mentioned stained the collagen yellow and showed fine collagen fibres which in some cases enclosed the superficial or deeper deposits.

2. *Masson's trichrome:* the superficial lesions were stained blue, whereas the collagen stroma was stained unevenly red.

3. *Gomori's trichrome staining:* the superficial and deep areas were not stained.

4. *Wilder's method for reticulin:* all the collagen of the stroma was positive, as also were the fine fibrils enclosing the deposits. The deposits themselves were negative. Very positive fibrous or grumous debris could be observed, corresponding to the fragmented collagen in course of degeneration.

102

5. *Van Gieson*: The collagen structures of the stroma were stained bright red, but the superficial lesions showed no staining.

The areas showing a hyaline appearance, as well as the more superficial and smaller lesions, were in some cases stained yellow by the saturated picric acid of the fuchsin solution. However, we observed this effect in only two cases.

6. *Colloidal iron according to Rinehart and Abul-Haj (Figs. 39 and 40)*: All the deposits were highly positive and were stained intensely blue by this method, which is rather specific for the mucopolysaccharides.

The superficial areas displayed an uneven positivity. The zones of hyaline appearance were less positive (greenish staining). Some of these areas, smaller and more homogeneous, were taking the yellow colour of picric acid.

The granulations of the interlamellar deposits and those of the keratocyte cytoplasm had an identical appearance. They were stained dark blue, taking on the whole the appearance of caviar.

The collagen structures were stained red and the fine collagen fibres surrounding or enclosing the deposits were stained pink or yellow (by the picric acid of the fuchsin solution).

7. *Alcian blue (Figs. 41, 42, 43, 44 and 45)*: All the superficial, interlamellar and intracytoplasmic granular deposists were positive for Alcian blue at pH values between 1 and 8. The granulations were bright blue stained. The

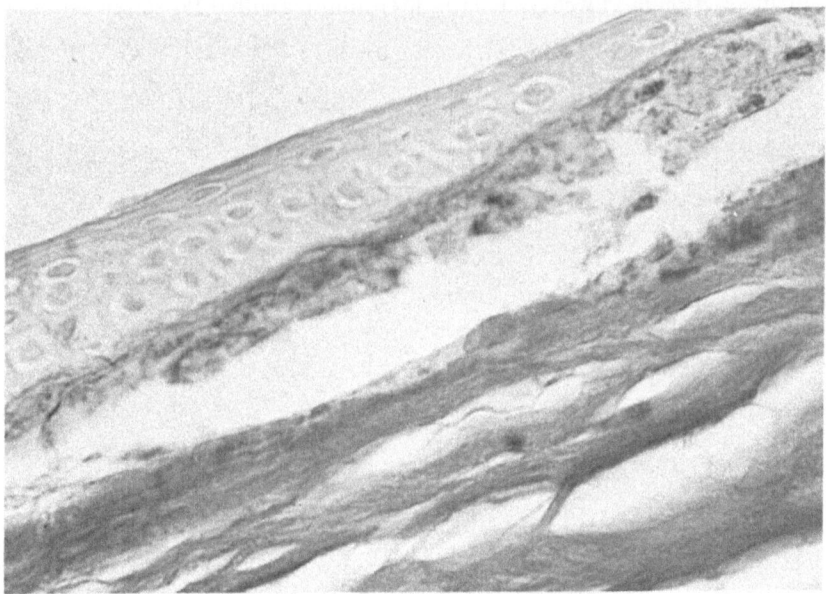

Fig. 39. Superficial area positive for mucopolysaccharides (blue). Rinehart and Abul-Haj staining (x 25 obj.).

superficial deposits displayed a less homogeneous positivity. The hyaline areas were less positive, whatever the pH value. The positivity of the lamellae was weaker than that of the deposits, but they were stained at the same pH values.

The critical saline concentration, capable of inhibiting the staining by Alcian blue, was that of 1.3 M magnesium chloride for pH 1 Alcian blue. Saline concentrations below 1.3 M magnesium chloride did not inhibit the staining by Alcian blue of pH 1 or more. We recall that magnesium chloride blocks the acid groups of the mucopolysaccharides, so that the more acid groups present, the higher the saline concentration necessary to neutralise them and to prevent the staining by Alcian blue.

8. *Metachromatic curves with toluidine blue.* The granules stored in the keratocytes, as well as those of the superficial and interlamellar deposits, displayed typically a strong metachromasia for all values of pH ranging from 0.5 or 1 to 8 or more. The metachromasia was of type β below pH 3, and of type γ above pH 3. The γ-metachromasia was red or pink, and the β-metachromasia more purplish blue.

9. *Staining with acridine orange after Saunder's method (1964). (Fig. 46)*, which consists in the simultaneous staining of three adjacent sections of the same series. The three sections were first treated with cetylpyridinium chloride and washed with tap water. They were next treated with ribonuclease. Finally, section no. 1 was treated for three minutes with 0.1% acridine orange.

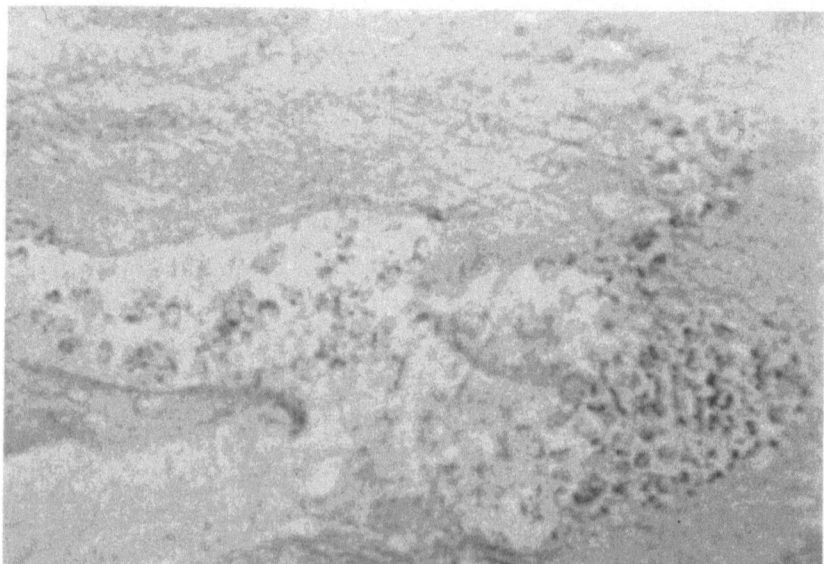

Fig. 40. Flat section. Mucopolysaccharidic granulations (blue). Rinehart and Abul-Haj staining (x 100 obj.).

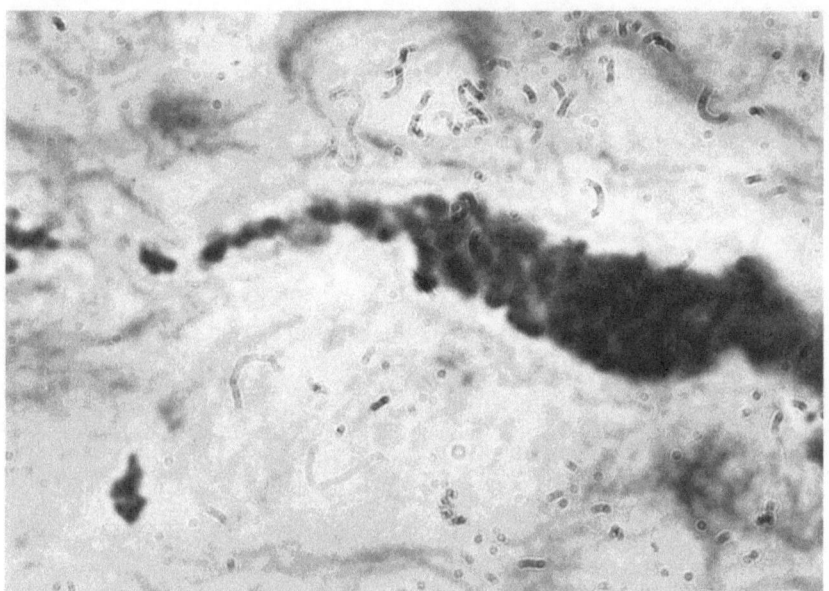

Fig. 41. Storage in a keratocyte. Highly positive mucopolysaccharidic granulations. 2.5 pH Alcian blue staining (x 100 obj.).

Section no. 2 was treated with pH 3.5 acridine orange and washed and differentiated in 0.3 M sodium chloride dissolved in 0.01 M acetic acid. Section No. 3 was treated as section no. 2, except that the 0.3 M sodium chloride was replaced by 0.6 M sodium chloride.

The granules of the keratocytes as well as the superficial and deep affected areas were stained in all three sections, because of the presence of highly sulphated mucopolysaccharides.

10. *Direct Schiff's reaction*, which indicates the presence of free aldehyde groups, was negative.

11. *Staining with periodic acid Schiff (PAS) (Fig. 47)*. We adopted two oxidation times: five and fifteen minutes. The positivity was very intense in the superficial areas, which were stained magenta red. In two cases, we found small, more homogeneous lesions which were stained positively, but more pink. The interlamellar deposits and the granules of the keratocytes were both as positive, but the staining was less intense than at the level of the superficial deposits.

On flat sections, extensive areas were seen, displaying granules which sometimes grouped in clots. These granules corresponded in part to those observed at the phase-contrast microscope. The extent of the PAS-positive area was, however, greater than that of the areas of granules previously localised at the phase-contrast microscope.

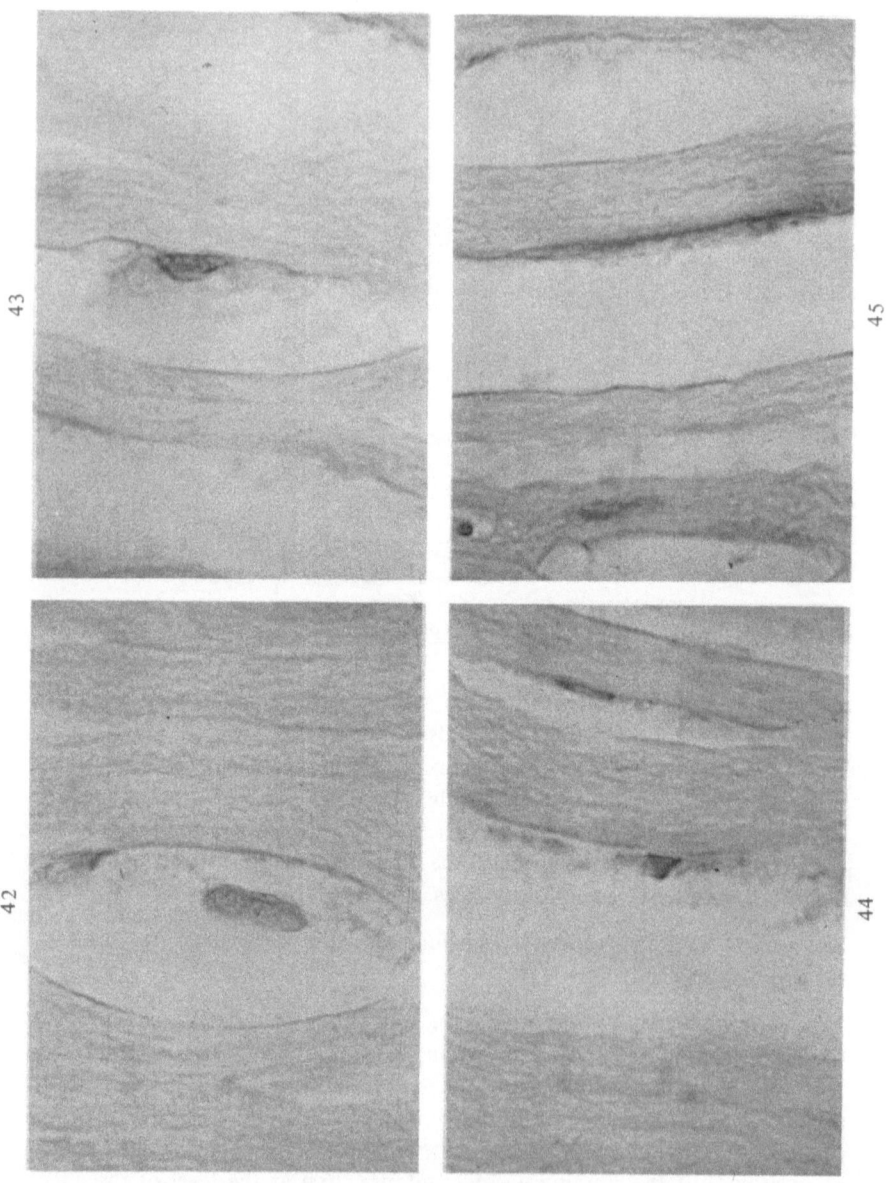

Various stages of the storage in the keratocytes (1 pH Alcian blue, staining x 100 obj.). The mucopolysaccharides are blue stained:

Fig. 42. Stage I. Normal nucleus.
Fig. 43. Stage II. Globular shape.
Fig. 44. Stage III. Pycnotic nucleus.
Fig. 45. Stage IV. The nucleus has disappeared. Only an interlamellar deposit remains.

12. *Toluidine blue in aluminium sulphate* gave a metachromatic staining in the superficial and deep areas, as well as in the granulations of the keratocytes.

13. *Nile blue* gave a blue staining to the superficial and deep areas, as well as to the cytoplasm of the keratocytes.

14. *Pyronine* stained the superficial and deep areas weakly red.

15. *Staining for lipids.* Oil Red 'O', Sudan III and Sudan black, as well as Schultze's reaction for cholesterol, were negative at the levels of all the lesions.

16. *Acridine orange after Mortelmans and Sebruyns.* The nuclei of the pathological keratocytes displayed a green fluorescence, in many cases masked by the red fluorescence of the cytoplasm. The nuclei were in the course of picnosis, for the fluorescence was distributed in clots. The cytoplasm displayed a fluorescence ranging from orange-yellow to red, which, however, was not totally due to RNA, since the ribonuclease test was negative.

17. *The stainings for amyloid* (Congo red, thioflavin 'T' and crystal violet) were all negative.

18. *Hyaluronidase test.* The prior treatment with bovine testicular hyaluronidase did not neutralize the metachromasia for toluidine blue, the colloidal-iron reaction or the stainings with Alcian blue or PAS.

19. *Takeuchi and Tanoue's method for acid phosphatase* (Figs. 48 and 49), which is a modification of Gomori's classical method. It was positive (staining ranging from brown to black) in the granular parts of the superficial areas of the stroma, in the granules of the keratocytes and in isolated granules of the corneal stroma. The granulations containing acid phosphatase were as a consequence intra- and extracellular.

20. The *standard azo-dye coupling* method for the detection of the acid phosphatases gave identical results to those of the Takeuchi and Tanoue method.

C. *Polarisation microscopy and topo-optical staining (Fig. 47)*

The granulations of the keratocytes and the interlamellar deposits were anisotropic. The round granules took on the configuration of a maltese cross, constituting so typical 'spherites'. These spherites were negative, as their birefringence was negative relative to their radius. The figures were nevertheless in many cases incomplete. After the phenol reaction, the sign of the collagen positive birefringence became negative, whereas that of the spherites remained unchanged.

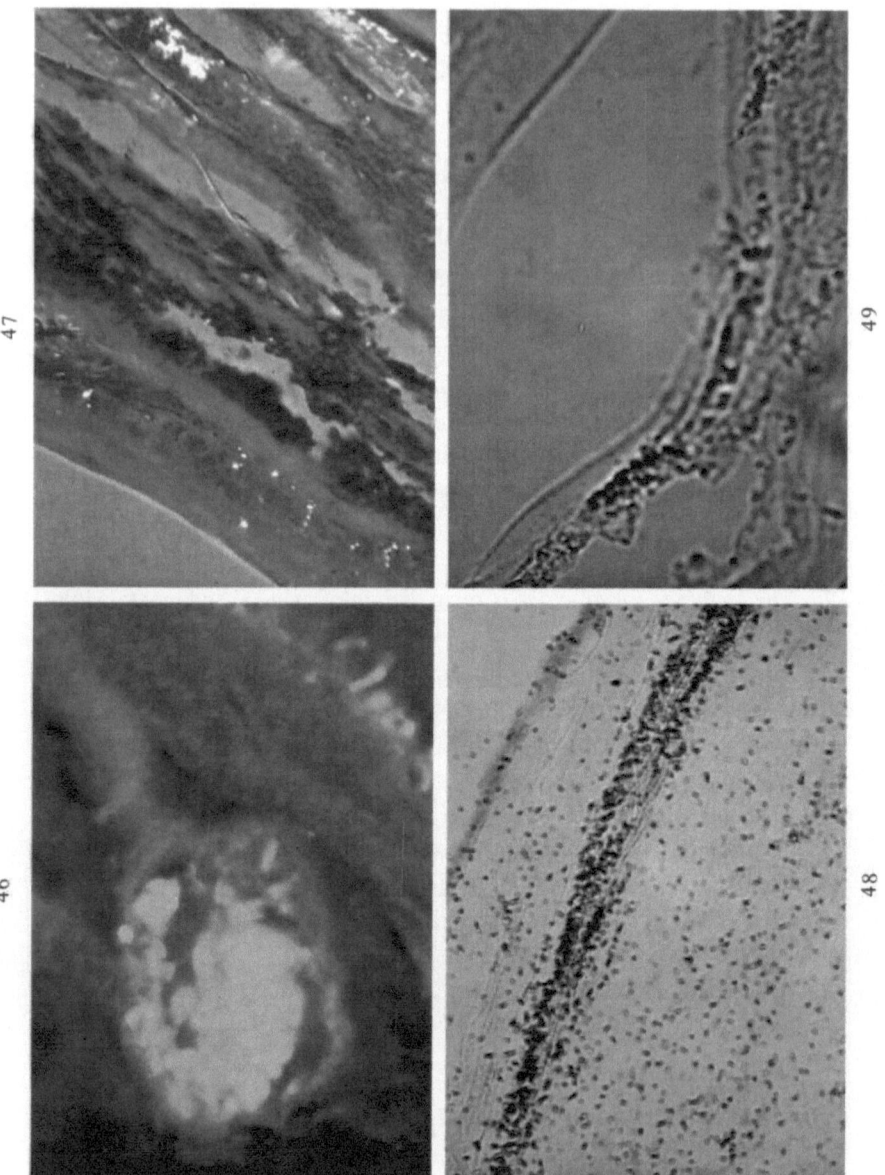

Fig. 46. Saunder's method. The keratosulphates in the keratocytes show an orangish fluorescence. Fluorescence microscopy (x 100 obj.).

Fig. 47. Very extensive superficial area containing positive material. The collagen is birefringent. PAS staining. Polarisation microscopy (x 25 obj.).

Fig. 48. Acid phosphatases according to Takeuchi and Tanoue method. The stromal lesions are positive (brown deposits) (x 25 obj.).

Fig. 49. At greater magnification, acid phosphastases (black) in the granulations (x 100 obj.).

After staining with PAS, Alcian blue (pH 2.5) and colloidal iron, the birefringence of the granules diminished. After staining the sections with topo-optical dyes (rivanol and precipitation with potassium ferrocyanide, followed by staining with toluidine blue), the birefringence of the spherites increased.

The anisotropy varied from one granule to another.

The granules positive for the histochemical dyes of mucopolysaccharides, had a much weaker birefringence after staining.

The lesions of the superficial stroma, which were stained yellow by the Van Gieson picric acid and colloidal iron, pale pink by PAS and blue by the Masson trichrome (two cases), displayed the following characteristics.

The birefringence was negative after mounting both in Canada balsam and in arabic-gum. After staining with rivanol or toluidine blue, the birefringence increased only slightly and in any case, only half as much as that of normal collagen.

There were areas of corneal collagen, of apparently normal appearance at the optical microscope and after histochemical staining, which displayed a very substantial diminution and in some cases, even an absence of birefringence. The phenol reaction further reduced the birefringence or caused it even to disappear completely, instead of changing its sign.

Many collagen lamellae had a perfectly normal appearance at the polarisation microscope, both before and after topo-optical staining. It was in the depth that the largest number of normal lamellae was found. The interfibrillar oedema in many cases dissociated the collagen fibres.

D. Dark-field microscopy

This examination gave the most information, when sections stained with Alcian blue or, better still, with colloidal iron were examined. Changes could be seen in sections stained by Wilder's method.

a. *Sections stained with Alcian blue.* The pictures observed were similar whatever the pH value. The granulations of the interlamellar deposits and of the keratocytes appeared as particles which were either very bright and gold-coloured or in some cases black. In other cases, a gold-coloured sphere with a black spot in the centre could be seen. Such granules were found in the superficial areas, which had a polychrome appearance.

A characteristic feature was the presence, in the lamellae that appeared normal at the optical microscope, of polychrome, green or yellow coloured streaks. They had the appearance of needles oriented longitudinally in the lamellae. In some cases, parallel lines of polychrome specks were observed in the lamella. This appearance was not found in sections of normal corneas. This observation showed that the dark-field microscope revealed lesions earlier than other microscopical methods.

When these lamellae were examined alternately at the polarisation microscope and the dark-field microscope, it was seen that the polychrome lesions, observed on the dark field, displayed the loss of birefringence that we described above.

By using UV lighting and examining on the dark-field, the granules appeared bright blue.

b. *Sections stained with colloidal iron according to Rinehart and Abul-Haj.* The granulations had a silver-blue staining and were very bright, both at the level of the keratocytes and at that of the interlamellar deposits. Inside the collagen lamellae also, lines of polychrome granules and needles were found, which gave the lamellae red stained by the fuchsin a granular or filamentous appearance. As in the case of Alcian blue, the arrangement of the polychrome elements was longitudinal relative to the collagen fibres. The polychromia varied from yellow to pink.

On flat sections, the keratocytes, with their granulations, their pseudopodia and their eccentric nuclei, were very well visible.

When UV lighting and dark-field were used, only bright blue granules were seen.

c. *Sections stained by Wilder's method.* All the lamellae had a very bright gilded appearance. The degenerating collagen fragments, which displayed a more positive staining than the normal lamellae, when observed on a bright background, displayed at the dark-field a distinctly brighter gilded appearance. The clots of collagen consisted of specks and very closely packed small needles.

DISCUSSION AND CONCLUSIONS

From our observations it may be concluded that essentially lesions of five types are found.

1. Subepithelial areas, some with granular and others with more hyalinised zones. These areas are positive for sulphated mucopolysaccharides. The surrounding collagen is frayed and deteriorated.

2. Storage granules in the keratocytes. They are also positive for sulphated mucopolysaccharides.

3. Interlamellar deposits of identical granules.

4. Small areas in the anterior stroma, stained yellow by the picric acid of the fuchsin of Rinehart and Abul-Haj or Van Gieson. These areas display negative birefringence at the polarisation microscope. The birefringence of this material does not change when either arabic gum is added or after the phenol reaction. The topo-optical dyes increase the birefringence only very

slightly. It can, therefore, be concluded that these lesions do not contain mucopolysaccharides and that they have only the topo-optical characteristics of collagen. According to François et al. (1972c), it is a material arranged transversely between the collagen fibres and constituting dense basophilic structures.

5. The collagen lamellae, which at the optical microscope have a seemingly normal appearance after histochemical staining, but which are seen to be damaged at the polarisation or dark-field microscope. The deterioration consists, on the one hand, in a reduction of the birefringence and, on the other hand, in the rupture of polychrome elements, when the sections are stained with Alcian blue and colloidal iron.

The stored granules display positive reactions for mucopolysaccharides. Their characteristics are the following:

1. They are already visible at the phase-contrast microscope. Unlike the granules of Kitano (1966, 1969), they are seen equally well in the sections fixed with fixatives that do not contain cetylpyridinium chloride. This fact indicates that the mucopolysaccharides of the granules are not soluble.

2. The granules are not eosinophil.

3. The granules apparently do not contain precursors of mature collagen, because the Wilder and Van Gieson stainings are negative, as well as the polarisation microscopy.

4. The granules are very positive for colloidal iron. However, this staining does not inform us as to which polyanions are linked with the iron ions (Fe^{++}).

5. Alcian blue stains the granules, whatever the pH value. This fact shows that, with a very acid value of pH, free negative charges are still found, capable of linking with the dye.

Moreover, the critical saline concentrations with magnesium chloride show that a very high molarity is necessary to inhibit a positive staining with Alcian blue, even higher than that necessary to neutralise the staining of the lamellae. Staining with Alcian blue at very acid pH values and a high critical saline concentration are characteristic of the sulphated polyanions.

6. The metachromatic curve for toluidine blue shows a metachromatic staining of the granules at very acid pH values. This curve is characteristic of the sulphated mucopolysaccharides (keratosulphate).

7. Saunder's method using acridine orange also gives a positivity characteristic of the sulphated mucopolysaccharides.

8. The negative direct Schiff and the positive PAS staining indicate that the oxidation by periodic acid liberates a large number of aldehydes at the level of the mucopolysaccharide chains. This liberation is very rapid; it is already complete after five minutes of oxidation.

9. Nile blue and toluidine blue in aluminium sulphate stain the granules positively.

10. The enzymatic test of neutralisation with hyaluronidase is negative, which excludes the presence of sulphated or unsulphated hyaluronic acid and of chrondroitin sulphate A and C, these mucopolysaccharides being sensitive to hyaluronidase.

11. The granules appear not to contain RNA, when the Mortelmans and Sebruyns method is applied, the ribonuclease test being apparently negative. Some of the granules are nevertheless positive for pyronine, a reagent which indicates the presence of RNA. The positivity of the ribonuclease test might be masked by the presence of insoluble mucopolysaccharides, when the dye is acridine orange.

12. The granules contain acid phosphatase, which indicates the lysosomal origin of the granules, as the particles positive for acid phosphatase cannot be other than primary or secondary lysosomes. If they are secondary, they can also contain mucopolysaccharides or even phagocyted particles.

13. At the polarisation microscope, it is observed that the granules display oriented structures of the 'spherite' type (François et al., 1972c). These structures are oriented concentrically, but incompletely. The orientation is laminated, but the arrangement is more irregular than in myelin (François et al., 1972c). The anisotropy of the granules is different from that characteristic of collagen. Moreover, the diminution of birefringence after staining for mucopolysaccharides indicates that this birefringence is due to the presence of polyanionic structures and, in addition, the topo-optical stainings indicate that those polyanionic structures are oriented.

The lesions around the mucopolysaccharide deposits involve the collagen fibres and the interstitial matrix. The changes of the apparently normal collagen lamellae display a deep deterioration of the intercellular corneal stroma.

In conclusion, granules containing highly sulphated insoluble mucopoly-saccharides and having the characteristics of keratosulphate are stored. These mucopolysaccharides are oriented and are probably arranged in irregular concentric sheets. The behaviour of the stored granules is in most of the cases that of secondary lysosomes, as they contain, in addition to the mucopolysaccharides, acid phosphatase and probably other lysosomal enzymes. The interlamellar and superficial lesions appear to be secondary to the breaking up of the keratocytes. There are also intralamellar lesions at the level of the collagen/interstitial-matrix complex. The impairment of the corneal sensitivity might theoretically be due to the presence, around the nerve, of pathological keratocytes or of deposits secondary to cellular ruptures.

CHAPTER VIII

TRANSMISSION ELECTRON MICROSCOPY OF THE CORNEAL STROMA IN MACULAR DYSTROPHY OF THE CORNEA

PERSONAL OBSERVATIONS

We shall describe the several stages in the keratocyte degeneration, as well as the extracellular stromal lesions.

A. Superficial layers of the corneal stroma

In the cases that we have examined, we have only rarely found a part of the Bowman's membrane to be normal or even present, outside the corneal periphery. When it existed, it was dissociated in fine, matted fibrils. The diameters of these fibrils were less than those of the corneal lamellae. Rounded clear spaces, which were only rarely delimited by a membrane, where found among the matted fibrils. These lesions represented a fibrillar and vacuolar degeneration of the membrane. It should be noted that keratocytes were always found in the vicinity.

In some cases, fragments of electron-dense collagen were seen.

In some places, small areas could be observed consisting of a material having the appearance of hyalin and an electron density similar to that of the base membrane of the epithelium.

In one case, the matted fine fibrils were located at a greater depth and were partially invaded by pathological keratocytes. It was due to a proliferation of collagen between the epithelium and the Bowman's membrane.

B. Keratocytes

It was possible to find in the same cornea the various stages of the keratocyte degeneration, although all the keratocytes displayed changes due to the storage, whether they be located in the superficial or in the deep layers of the stroma (Figs. 50, 51, 52 and 53).

I. First stage of the keratocyte degeneration

The following changes could be observed in the nucleus and the cytoplasm:
1. Hypertrophy of the Golgi's apparatus, with increase in the number of vacuoles, originating from the cisterns.
2. Dilation of the cisterns of the endoplasmic reticulum.

113

3. Presence of numerous particles of lysosomal type, whose contents had various electron densities.
4. Mitochondria of normal appearance, or in some cases dilated, with erased crests.
5. Intact cellular membrane.
6. Cells with numerous pseudopodia.

II. Second stage of the keratocyte degeneration

The nucleus showed a fragmented chromatin, the fragments adhering to the nuclear membrane.

The cytoplasm had greatly increased in volume. It displayed a denser cytoplasmic matrix with some tonofibrils and some membrane debris. It contained the following elements:

a. *Particles of lysosomal type.*
1. Particles of lysosomal type with no electron density and in appearance empty, measuring from 0.5 to 0.8 μm and having a well-defined membrane.
2. Larger elements than the foregoing, measuring between 1 and 3 μm,

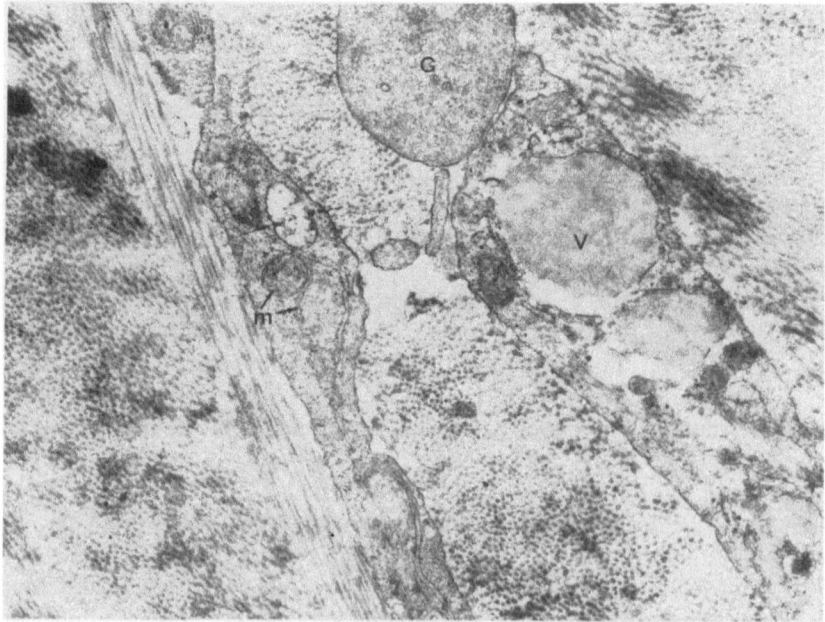

Fig. 50. Keratocyte with large vacuoles (V) containing a finely fibrillar electron-dense material. (M) mitochondria. (G) large extracellular vacuoles containing a finely granular material. Transmission electron microscopy (x 7500).

114

more numerous, probably formed by the fusion of the preceding particles and surrounded by a complete membrane.

3. Particles of lysosomal type containing a finely granulated material of low electron density. Their dimensions were variable, but rather large (more than 1.5 μm). Their membranes were complete.

4. Rounded elements of lysosomal type, containing a velvety material of fairly high electron density. Their membranes were well-defined. There was a very narrow (120 Å) clear space between the contents of the particle and its membrane.

5. Lysosomes having the same appearance as the preceding particles, but only half or quarter filled, the remainder of the intralysosomal space appearing to be empty.

6. Large lysosomes of 2 to 4 μm, formed by a single unit membrane enclosing a denser fibrillar or granular material. Within there was a rounded corpuscle of about 1 μm, also surrounded by a membrane and containing a denser material, in which specks of higher electron density were seen.

7. Lysosomes having the same characteristics as the foregoing, but without membrane around the enclosed corpuscle.

8. Lysosomes having the same appearance as the foregoing, but in which

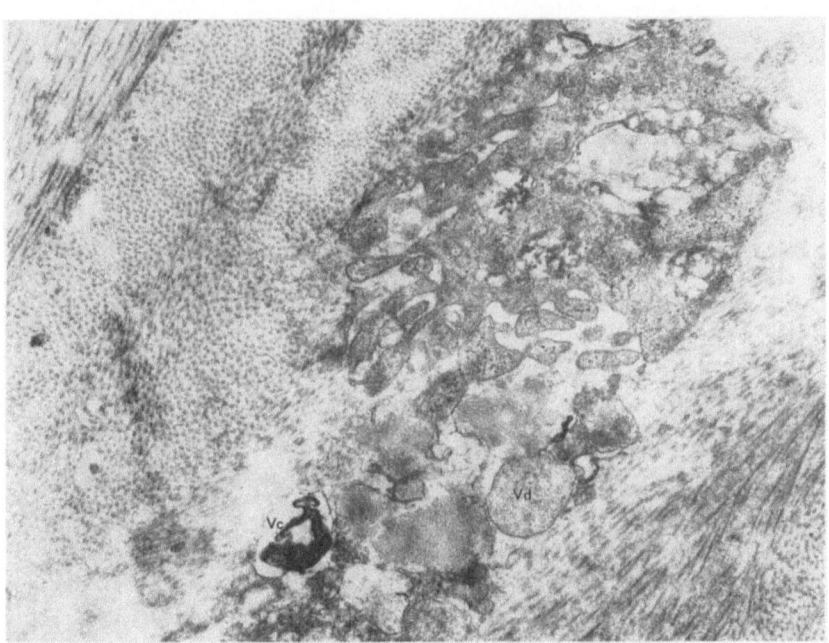

Fig. 51. Rupture of a keratocyte and reconstruction after discharge of some vacuoles. (Vd) vacuoles containing electron-dense material. (Vc) vacuole containing cell debris. Transmission electron microscopy (× 7625).

the inner corpuscle was represented by a complete or fragmented membrane constituted by a crown of very electron-dense clumps. They appeared to be empty.

9. Multivesicular bodies formed by a membrane enclosing a matrix of variable electron density and in which five or six apparently empty vesicles were observed.

10. Lysosomes surrounded by a well-defined membrane, and having contents of moderate electron density, which showed clearer and finer (50 Å) longitudinal striations. In some cases, the arrangement of these striations was more radiate, relative to the lysosomal sphere, but there was always a certain parallelism between them.

These lysosomes, which could also be found in the pseudopodia, might fuse. When their membrane was ruptured, the material tended to retain its shape, although it could also be found irregularly distributed in the cytoplasmic matrix.

11. In the extremities of the pseudopodia, small vesicles could be found. They did not exceed 0.1 μm, and their contents displayed variable electron densities.

12. Autophagic vesicles containing the membrane debris of the endoplasmic reticulum or of the mitochondria.

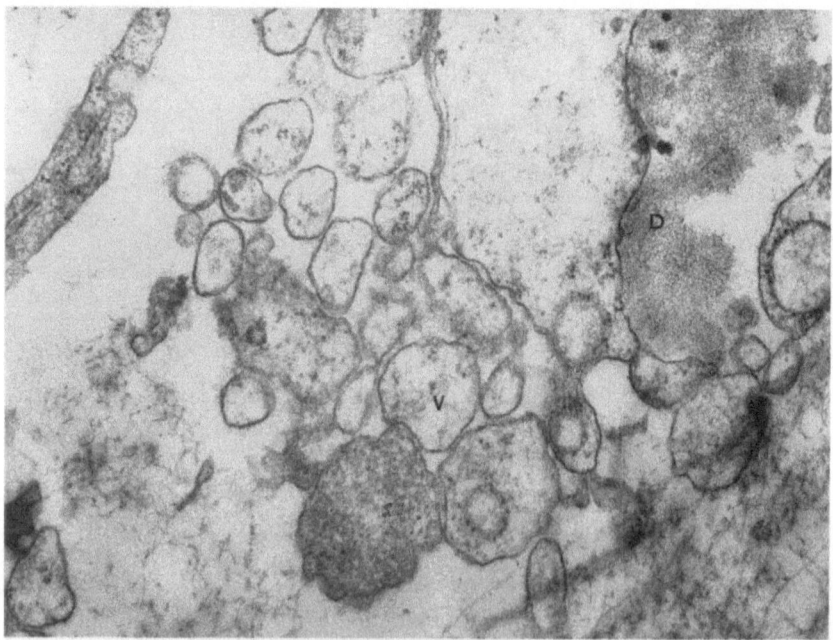

Fig. 52. Keratocyte after rupture of the cell membrane. (V) vacuoles filled with granular material. (D) deposits of electron-dense material. Transmission electron microscopy (x 13 875).

13. Two vesicles, one enclosed within the other. The membrane of the outer vesicle was partially fused with that of the inner vesicle.

14. Elements of irregular shape. Their contents had a very high electron density and consisted of a material of membranous origin.

15. Vesicles of various dimensions surrounded by double membranes and containing a granulo-fibrillar material of low electron density.

16. Lysosomes of 1 to 2 μm, containing a finely granular material with some spots of high electron density. In some cases, the lysosomal matrix showed at its centre a corpuscle of very high electron density, which was not surrounded by a membrane.

b. *Mitochondria.* Already at this stage, the mitochondria, less in number, showed some changes. The following types could be found:

1. Clear and dilated mitochondria, the crests of their interior membrane being erased.

2. Small mitochondria, with electron-dense contents and disorganised crests.

3. Mitochondria, with irregular electron density and deteriorated crests.

4. Mitochondria of normal appearance.

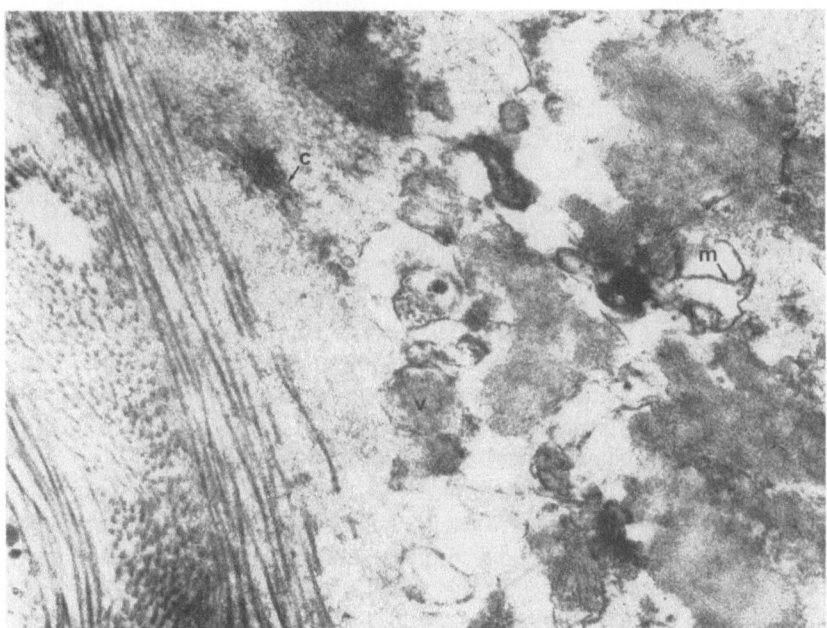

Fig. 53. After rupture of the cell, membrane debris (m), vacuoles (V) and a material of variable electron density can be observed. The collagen (c) is digested by enzymes liberated in the deposits. Transmission electron microscopy (x 11250).

We have not observed any merging of the degenerating mitochondria which were found inside the autophagic vesicles.

c. *Endoplasmic reticulum.* The cisterns of the endoplasmic reticulum, whether granular (with ribosomes) or agranular, were dilated and fused partially or wholly with the lysosomal membrane. Their contents displayed the following characteristics:
1. Material formed by filaments of moderate electron density and arranged as a meshwork, the cross-over points having a higher electron density.
2. Rolled up membrane debris.
3. Striated electron-dense material, which was also seen in the lysosomes.
4. In some cases, the ergastoplasmic cisterns appeared to be empty, although dilated.

d. *Golgi's apparatus.* When it could be identified, the Golgi's apparatus showed a hypertrophic appearance, characterised above all by the presence of a large number of membranous vesicles surrounding the cisterns, which were enlarged.

e. *Cellular membrane.* To the extent that it was possible to follow its path, it had not yet ruptured, all the elements described above being still intracellular.

III. Third stage of the keratocyte degeneration

At this stage, the cell membrane was ruptured and the pathological structures were in direct contact with the surrounding stroma. At some places, however, it was observed that, after the escape of a certain number of vesicles, the membrane was regenerated and partially recovered the cytoplasm, which still contained the pathological elements.

During this third stage, the usual appearance of the keratocyte was as follows. The cell membrane was ruptured and lacking over more or less extensive parts of the cell contour. In some cases, fragments of the ruptured cellular membrane could be seen, their structure as a membrane unit being still recognisable. Sometimes a central space was found, filled with a filamentous substance arranged as a meshwork and surrounded by lysosomal, ergastoplasmic or mixed vesicles, as seen in the second stage.

In other cases still, a large striated area of electron-dense material was observed, with membrane debris, enclosing it segmentarily. These areas were also surrounded by vesicles and lysosomes, some of which were open toward the striated material. Between the vesicles there might be a filamentous material.

IV. Fourth and final stage of the keratocyte degeneration

During this stage, the vesicles and the various materials described above constituted a real interfascicular deposit. The vesicles of different diameters were dispersed and invaded the whole parenchyme. In one and the same area might be found:
1. Rounded lysosomes with velvety contents, having still a well-defined membrane.
2. Free velvety material.
3. Striated material of electron density similar to or greater than that of the velvety material.
4. Lysosomes of various types, surrounded by a membrane and having variable contents.
5. A loose fibrous meshwork, located between the disseminated elements and the neighbouring collagen.
6. Cytoplasmic debris containing fragments of the endoplasmic reticulum and numerous electron-dense particles.
7. Vesicles having a highly electron-dense and greatly thickened membrane, which could nevertheless be ruptured.

C. INTERCELLULAR CORNEAL STROMA

In numerous places, the stroma showed interfascicular deposits, which corresponded to the keratocytes in the final stage of thesaurismosis. We were able to find the following deposits, either isolated or grouped:
1. Areas of electron-dense material which was in some places velvety and in others striated. This material was of the same type as that seen in the cells. The deposits were connected with the neighbouring collagen, which they appeared to invade. When the striated material was examined at the densitometer, it was seen that the striae had a very uniform periodicity. Each stria measured 140 Å, and the distance between two striae was 160 Å. These figures recalled the microperiodicity of the collagen.
2. Very fine filaments of about 180 Å arranged in a meshwork. In many cases they sourrounded the degenerating keratocyte. They united the collagen fibres by constituting a meshwork, whose cross-over points were formed by the transversely directed collagen fibrils.
3. Highly electron-dense areas consisting of stromal collageñ fibrils. In many cases there was a densification, so that the collagen striation was only seen in some places. This material was not always connected with the degenerated keratocytes.

These areas and the filaments showed the same characteristics as those that we saw inside the keratocytes.

Large clear spaces, formed by the merging of vesicles, were also seen in the stroma. In places, the divisions between the vesicles could still be seen, so that the whole had the appearance of honey-combs.

DISCUSSION AND CONCLUSIONS

In general, our observations concerning the superficial layers of the corneal stroma are in concordance with those of Teng (1966), Hermann et al. (1971), Snip et al. (1973), François et al. (1974b and 1975a).

It seems that the Bowman's membrane becomes fibrillar, since the fibrils, constituting the superficial collagen matting, are finer than the fibres of the deep stroma.

Our observations on the keratocytes agree also with those of other authors (Klintworth et al., 1964; Offret et al., 1966; Morgan, 1966; Teng, 1966; Thiel et al., 1971; Hermann et al., 1971; Malbran, 1972; Blümcke et al., 1972; Malbran et al., 1973; Snip et al., 1973; François et al., 1974b and 1975a).

The intracytoplasmic vacuoles have a variable content: fibrillar, electron-dense with or without striation, finely granular, etc. Some other vacuoles appear to be empty.

There is a close relationship between the particles of lysosomal type and the cisterns of the endoplasmic reticulum. Fusion between the membranes of these two structures is, indeed, observed, with the result that the large vesicular spaces are derived from both the lysosomes and the endoplasmic reticulum. Such fusions, moreover, have been observed in other storage diseases (Heers et al., 1973).

The striated areas are very characteristic and probably represent the birefringent material of the cytoplasmic granules described by François et al. (1972c). When that material, which has a laminated structure, invades the collagen, the latter may take on a birefringence, the sign of which is not reversed by rivanol.

The transmission electron microscope shows that there is a progressive accumulation of vacuoles and of stored material until the cell ruptures.

The vacuoles of lysosomal type probably explain the positive histochemical reactions for mucopolysaccharides and acid phosphatase. However, in view of the fact that the soluble mucopolysaccharides are not electron-dense, these vacuoles mostly appear to be empty. The mucopolysaccharides can probably either become linked with a dense matrix, or remain free, as in the case of Kitano's granules.

The hypertrophy of the Golgi's apparatus is extremely important, because it synthesises the mucopolysaccharides and forms the intracellular membranes.

Our observations concerning the extracellular corneal stroma agree with these of Teng (1966), Offret et al. (1966), Hermann et al. (1971), Malbran

120

(1972), Malbran et al. (1973), François et al. (1975a). Other authors (Klint-worth et al., 1972), on the contrary, found no changes of the collagen stroma. By the way we may recall that François et al. (1972c) observed evident changes of the collagen at the polarisation microscope: on the one hand, a loss of birefringence in the areas of apparently normal collagen, and, on the other hand, changes of probably non-collagen structures.

We are able to confirm the results of François et al., (1972c) and to add the following:

1. There are changes of the lamellae, which are evidenced by the histo-chemical stainings and at the dark-field microscope.

2. There are fragments of collagen which are much more positive for Wilder's staining than normal collagen.

3. At the transmission electron microscope, areas are found where the collagen is very electron-dense, the fibrils occupying a matrix which is also more electron-dense than normally.

These various changes observed by different methods might well correspond to lesions of the same type.

We were able to identify real collagen fibres in the keratocytes. Nevertheless, we do not know the origin of the fine fibrils constituting the matted areas. They might be filaments of collagen, deteriorated by the liberation of lysosomal collagenase, which, indeed, can break up the collagen fibres. The fragments would then be phagocyted by the keratocytes, since, as we were able to demonstrate 'in vitro', the pathological keratocytes in tissue culture retain their normal capacity of phagocytosis.

The last two stages of the keratocyte degeneration give rise to interlamellar deposits, which we observed microscopically after histochemical stainings.

Our observations at the electron microscope are complementary to our histochemical observations. From the morphological point of view, we may conclude:

1. The keratocytes display numerous particles of lysosomal type, large dilated cisterns, and vacuoles that are either empty or contain a various material, which progressively accumulates until the cell bursts.

2. The material released by the cells acts on the neighbouring stroma, which degenerates.

3. There is a close relationship between the stromal changes and the keratocytes. Indeed, the areas of degenerated stroma, always contain a degenerating keratocyte. We have never observed an isolated lesion of the stroma.

CHAPTER IX

SCANNING ELECTRON MICROSCOPY OF THE CORNEAL STROMA IN MACULAR DYSTROPHY

PERSONAL OBSERVATIONS

We were able to study at the scanning electron microscope a cornea affected by macular dystrophy. In order to expose the corneal stroma, we proceeded in two different ways:

a. by making an opening in the posterior limiting membrane;

b. by cutting the cornea very obliquely, so as to expose the maximum of surface.

We were able to observe the following changes:

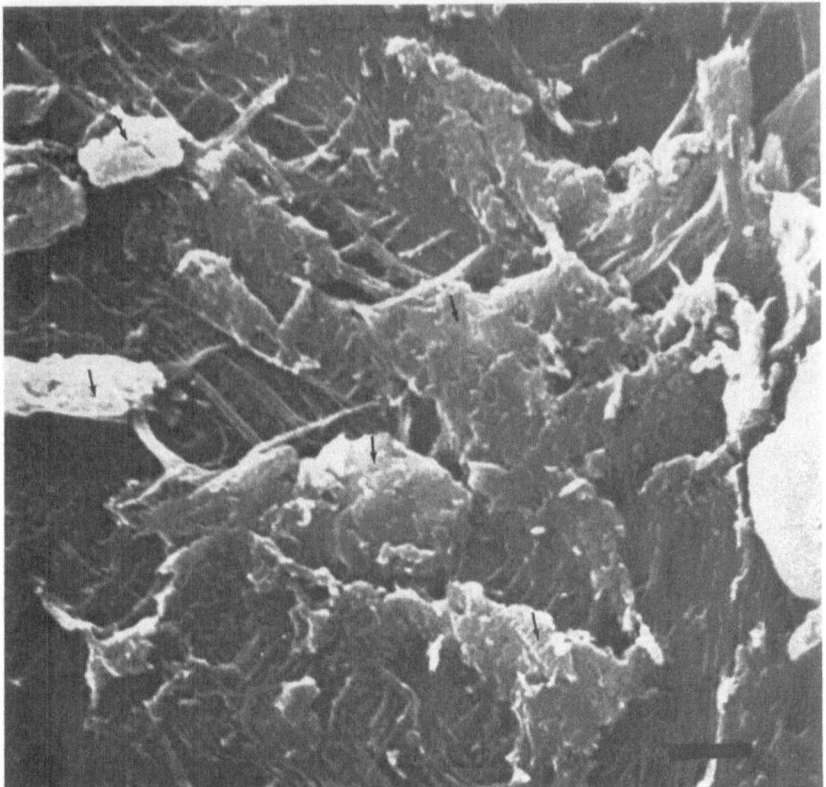

Fig. 54. Through a posterior opening, collagen fibres and fascicles can be observed. Some globular deposits (arrow) are also seen. Scanning electron microscopy (x 1412).

1. When the stroma was observed through a posterior opening, it showed a normal architectonic. The layers of collagen fascicles crossed one another at an angle of 45°. However, some irregular deposits might be seen in the deepest part of the opening (Fig. 54). In some cases, globular keratocytes adhering to the collagen structures were found. They were polymorphic and their surface was very irregular. Their longest axis measured from 3 to 15 μm.

2. The obliquely cut corneas showed that the lamellae deeply located displayed multiple deposits of polymorphic appearance, of 1.5 to 8 μm (Fig. 55). Their appearance was either granular or grumous.

    The accumulation of this material was in many cases more abundant between the last collagen lamella and the Descemet's membrane. The intermediate lamellae were more tightly packed, and for that reason, the granular deposits were less visible and smaller, measuring about 2.3 μm.

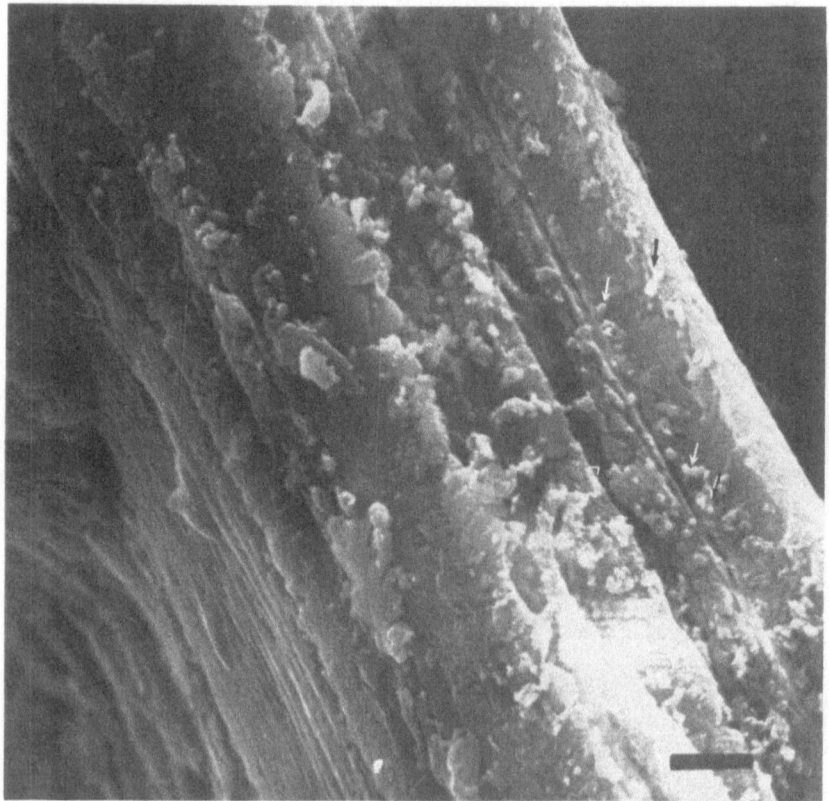

Fig. 55. From top to bottom, the endothelium, the Descemet's membrane with deposits (arrows) and the deep lamellae invaded by granulations can be observed. Scanning electron microscopy (x 692).

The superficial part of the stroma was occupied by large granular deposits. On an average the granulations measured 1.3 μm. They were very tightly packed (Fig. 56) and disorganized the lamellae.

CONCLUSION

The histochemical examination of the specimen, carried out at the same level as that seen at the scanning electron microscope, shows that the various granular deposits seen in all the stromal layers, consist of a mucopolysaccharide material.

The scanning electron microscope evidences the severe deterioration of the stromal architectonic. It shows the invasion and destruction of the collagen fascicles by the granular material, as well as the invasion of the posterior layers and the interposition of a finely granular material between the last collagen lamella and the Descemet's membrane.

As we have already said, this granular material consists of mucopolysaccharides and in particular of keratosulphate.

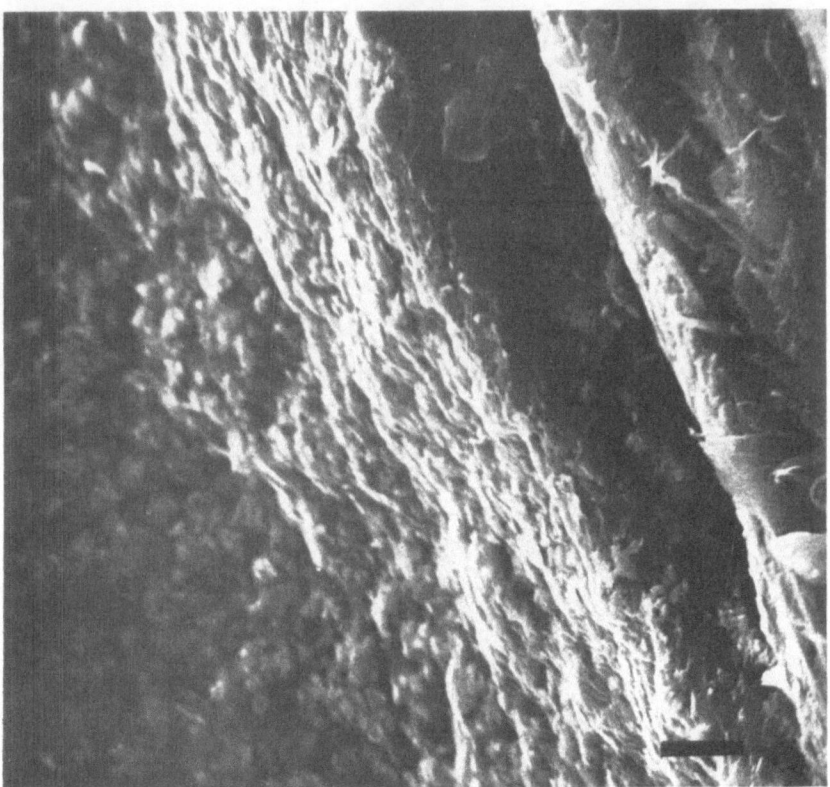

Fig. 56. Large superficial deposit formed by a granular material. The lamellae are dissected by the granules. Scanning electron microscopy (x 692).

CHAPTER X

CHANGES OF THE EPITHELIUM, THE BASE MEMBRANE, THE ENDOTHELIUM AND THE DESCEMET'S MEMBRANE IN MACULAR DYSTROPHY OF THE CORNEA

PERSONAL OBSERVATIONS

I. DETERIORATION OF THE EPITHELIUM AND THE BASE MEMBRANE

A. *Optical microscopy and histochemistry*

a. Examination at the clear-field microscope of stained sections

1. Staining with *haemotoxylin-eosin-saffron* showed the irregularity of the corneal epithelium. It was reduced to one or two cellular layers, when it covered the large superficial stromal lesions.

The epithelium as a whole was disorganised. Very thin parts could be seen, alongside parts of normal thickness. The basal layer was irregular, and proliferated into the stroma. There were areas with desquamation of the superficial cells.

Where the base membrane was lacking, the stromal cells could reach the basal cells and even migrate between the epithelial cells. These cells were generally flattened and undulated, showing large basophil nuclei.

Among the epithelial cells with strongly basophil nuclei, there were others with picnotic nuclei. This appearance was more evident in flat sections, 4 to 6 μm thick.

The cellular eosinophilia was reduced by an intracellular oedema. It was, indeed, possible to find areas with clearer basal cells and others with red-pink cells showing a normal eosinophilia.

2. When *Fast Red* was used as nuclear dye, the changes of the nuclei were even more evident.

3. *Wilder's method* for reticulin indicated the following changes:
a. The proportion of Teng's cells was increased. There were very dense cells, whose cytoplasm was strongly positive. They were polygonal and displayed short extensions, which gave them a stellar appearance.
b. The intercellular spaces were filled with a positive granular substance identical to that which filled the cytoplasm of the Teng's cells.
c. The argyrophil component of the epithelial base membrane was lacking

127

in many cases. In some places, nevertheless, the membrane was represented by a well-defined line, while in others it consisted of a chain of fine granules, as if it was fragmented.

4. The *stainings for mucopolysaccharides* (colloidal iron according to Rinehart and Abul-Haj, pH 1 and pH 2.5 Alcian blue) had the following characteristics:
a. The positivity of the superficial keratinised layer was weak.
b. The fibroblastic cells which penetrated the epithelium, or neighboured its basal cells, were keratocytes storing mucopolysaccharide granules.

5. *Toluidine blue* merely confirmed the nuclear changes. The nuclei of the epithelial cells were orthochromatic and in many cases showed signs of picnosis.

6. *Periodic acid Schiff* (PAS) indicated the presence of PAS-positive granules in the basal and intermediate layers of the epithelium. They were irregular, in some cases grouped, and measured between 0.5 and 1.5 μm. At high magnification, they gave the impression that they consisted of free intracytoplasmic material, rather than of real granules. The staining was also positive in the keratinised cells of the superficial layer. The PAS-positive structures had a more marked positivity after fifteen minutes of oxidation by periodic acid. The PAS staining was negative in extensive areas of the base membrane, which could, however, be partly normal. Areas of small PAS-positive granules could also be seen, extending beyond the base membrane in order to form a real deposit. These very refringent granules measured about 0.5 μm.

7. The *direct Schiff reaction* was negative in the epithelial cells.

8. The *stainings for lipids* (Oil Red 'O', Sudan III and Sudan black) were also negative.

9. The *staining with acridine orange* according to Mortelmans and Sebruyns for the nucleic acids showed an orange-red fluorescence in the basal and intermediate layers. RNA was present in the cytoplasm, the oedema vacuoles being nevertheless optically empty. The nuclei displayed a green fluorescence, which was weaker in the picnotic nuclei. In some cases, nuclear fragments showing a green fluorescence were found.

10. The *Takeuchi and Tanoue staining for acid phosphatase* was positive in the small granulations of the basal epithelial layer and, to a lesser degree, in the intermediate layers. The superficial layers were negative.

b. Phase-contrast microscopy of
fresh or histochemically-stained sections.

This microscopy made possible a better visualisation of the vacuoles and of the intracellular or intercellular epithelial oedema.

In the case of *intracellular oedema*, a 'dilution' of the cytoplasmic dyes was observed. Eosin stained the cytoplasm more weakly. In addition, there was a vacuolisation of the cytoplasm. The vacuoles of the basal cells were larger than those of the intermediate layer. In some cases the whole of a cell could be occupied by a single vacuole containing nuclear and cytoplasmic debris. Other cells with normal or picnotic nuclei showed an areolar cytoplasm consisting of numerous small vacuoles. The oedematous cells moved and distorted the neighbouring elements. The intracytoplasmic vacuoles were weakly eosinophil and were not stained by other histochemical dyes.

The *intercellular oedema* was very marked. It was characterised by a dilation of the intercellular spaces because of the progressive break of the desmosomes, which attached these cells one to another. The following could be observed:
1. A large intercellular space divided up by cytoplasmic strings.
2. An intercellular space consisting of a chain of small 'vacuoles'.
3. A large rounded intercellular space, wherein the cells remained attached to the two extremities of the space. The cytoplasm and the nucleus of one of the cells were pressed back by the dilation of this space, whereas the cell took on an annular and its nucleus a flattened shape.
4. In the basal layer of the epithelium, there were pseudo-vacuoles between the basal cells and the Bowman's membrane or the corneal stroma. In some cases, the epithelial cells remained attached to the Bowman's membrane by two or three tight cytoplasmic strings.
5. In the superficial cells, intercellular spaces of pseudovacuolar appearance were also found, which explained why the cell detached progressively.

In the case of migration of keratocytes into the epithelium, they passed through the intercellular spaces, while remaining in contact with one of the cells.

c. Polarisation microscopy of
histochemically stained sections.

Anisotropy was found in the following structures:
1. The superficial cells which showed a positive birefringence, parallel to the longest axis of the cell, and displaying the characteristics of keratin, arranged in parallel sheets. The birefringence was bluish in the sections stained with colloidal iron or Alcian blue of pH 1 to 2.5. It was red in the sections stained with PAS.

2. Very fine anisotropic granules were also found in the basal cells.

3. The molecules of the tonofibrils stretched by the oedema vacuoles, were arranged in order to give a positive axial birefringence.

d. Dark-field microscopy of stained sections.

The cytoplasm showed innumerable small, polychromic and very closely packed granulations. Most of the intracellular vacuoles and all the intercellular pseudovacuoles were optically empty. Rounded, optically empty spaces were also observed between the basal cells and the stroma.

When sections stained by Wilder's method were examined, the base membrane consisted of gilded, very refringent granules measuring 0.5 μm. In the case of sections stained by PAS, the small PAS-positive granulations were very refringent and red in colour.

The superficial keratin layer consisted of very small (≈ 0.1 μm) granulations, bluish after staining with Alcian blue of pH 1 or 2.5 and with colloidal iron, reddish after staining with PAS. The PAS-positive areas found in the basal cell layer consisted of a very heterogeneous material containing red granulations of variable refringence and dimensions.

B. Transmission electron microscopy

In the *basal cells*, the cytoplasm consisted of a dense network of tonofibrils, the cytoplasmic matrix being granular. Numerous small cytoplasmic vesicles could be seen close to the cell membrane, touching the base membrane. There were also small membranous vesicles containing a homogeneous material of moderate electron density. These vesicles were rounded or irregular in shape, their membranes showing sometimes a high electron density. In the nucleus, a unit membrane was seen, surrounding irregular and very electron-dense chromatin specks in a clear caryoplasm. In many cases the desmosomes between the cells were ruptured. The intercellular space was normal or irregularly dilated. On each side of the cell membrane, clear spaces of vacuolar appearance could be found, containing sometimes cytoplasmic debris.

The *intermediate cells* displayed the same changes as the basal cells. Mostly a cytoplasmic vacuolisation close to the cell membrane and a rupture of the desmosomes were observed.

In the *superficial layer*, numerous liquefying cells were found, the nuclei being fragmented and the desmosomes ruptured. In some cases, fairly complete cells were breaking away.

However, the changes were much more marked in some more or less extensive areas, which consisted of basal and intermediate cells displaying the following features:

1. Some cells had a cytoplasmic matrix containing electron-dense granules and very numerous tonofibrils. These granules together with clear spaces could be grouped close to the nucleus. Nevertheless, a certain number of ribosomal ergastoplasmic membranes had a normal appearance. Between the nuclei and the tonofibrils, there were rounded formations consisting of concentrically arranged membranes. In the centre of these formations, electron-dense dots, similar to ribosomes and which were also seen disseminated throughout the cytoplasmic matrix, could be observed (Fig. 57).

The *nucleus* did not show any particular characteristic.

At the level of the intercellular spaces, numerous ruptured desmosomes were found. These spaces were enlarged and appeared to be empty or filled with an electron-dense granular material.

2. In this last case, the very active cells had highly developed reticulo-endoplasmic systems, consisting of numerous cisterns with clear contents. Their membranes contained numerous ribosomes. There were also electron-dense spots around the nucleus, the membrane of which was irregular.

3. In cells of this type, thick and very dense tonofibrils were distributed in the ectoplasmic part of the cytoplasm and formed a circular felt around the nucleus. Groups of very dense granules were also found. The endoplasm consisted of a matrix of medium density, containing numerous granules of

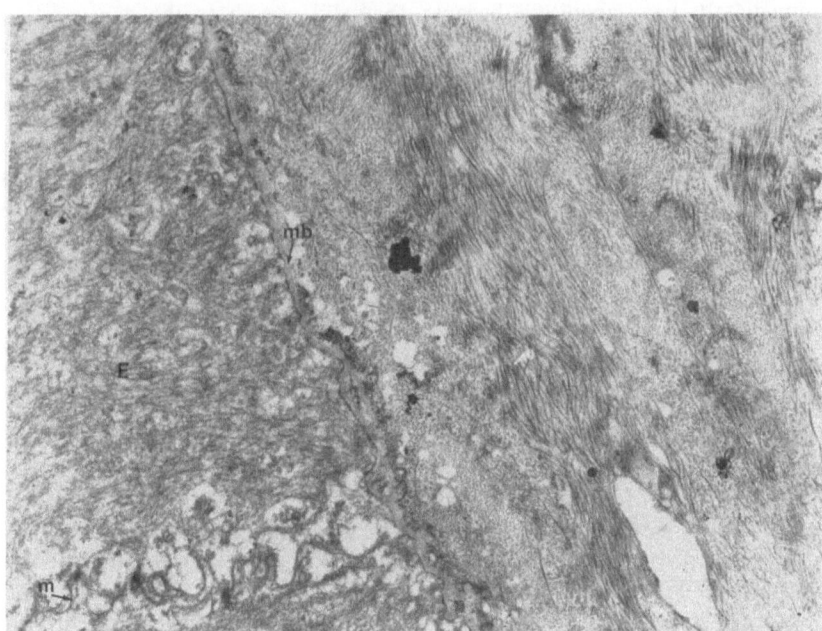

Fig. 57. (E) epithelial cell, (m) cell membrane. (mb) base membrane. The Bowman's membrane is replaced by stromal collagen. Transmission electron microscopy (x 7500).

the ribosomal type. In places, some vesicles of the lysosomal type were seen. At the level of the cellular membrane, clear spaces irregularly distributed were found.

4. In epithelial cells of another type, mostly located in the intermediate layer, the cytoplasmic matrix appeared to have shrunk.

An annular clear space existed around the nucleus, although clear spaces occurred also at the periphery. There were very dense and highly developed tonofibrils, which crossed one another at variable angles. They were arranged in the cytoplasmic matrix around the perinuclear clear halo. Debris of the matrix could adhere to the nuclear membrane. Some ergastoplasmic cisterns with ribosomes could be found. Small membranous vesicles and small mitochondria were observed here and there. The nucleus also was slightly shrunken. Its chromatin was distributed in large, highly electron-dense and irregular clumps. They were, indeed, pre-picnotic nuclei.

5. In two cases, we found epithelial cells, whose cytoplasm showed vacuolar spaces in a cytoplasmic matrix containing dense tonofibrils. These spaces were generally unique and were not surrounded by a membrane. They contained a finely filamentous and little electron-dense substance, surrounded by clear spaces.

Against the basal edge of the epithelial cells, or located between the epithelial cells of the basal layer, *macrophages* were also found. They could immediately be recognised, because they did not show the degeneration seen in the keratocytes, and because they did not contain densely packed tonofibrils, which differentiates them from the epithelial cells.

These cells had a very abundant cytoplasm. Their matrix consisted of a very loose granulo-filamentous meshwork, which contained a highly developed reticulo-endoplasmic system, formed of large cisterns filled with a material similar to that of the matrix. On the membranes of the macrophages, very numerous and mostly grouped ribosomes could be seen. Mitochondria of normal appearance and some vesicles of the lysosomal type, surrounded by a membrane and containing a granular material, were observed. The cells displayed some fine pseudopodia. There were vacuoles of pinocytosis close to the cellular membrane. The nucleus was irregular. Its chromatin was grouped and located against the cellular membrane, which consisted of a membrane unit, the two proteinic layers of which delimited a large clear lipidic space.

The *base membrane* of the epithelium showed more or less extensive interruptions. It consisted of a fine grey layer, measuring 0.2 to 0.5 μm.

Through the openings of the membrane, the cytoplasm of the adjacent epithelial cell extruded toward the stroma. There might also be irregular invaginations of the base membrane of the basal cell, which filled with the material constituting the base membrane.

In places, very electron-dense collagen fibrils originating from the de-

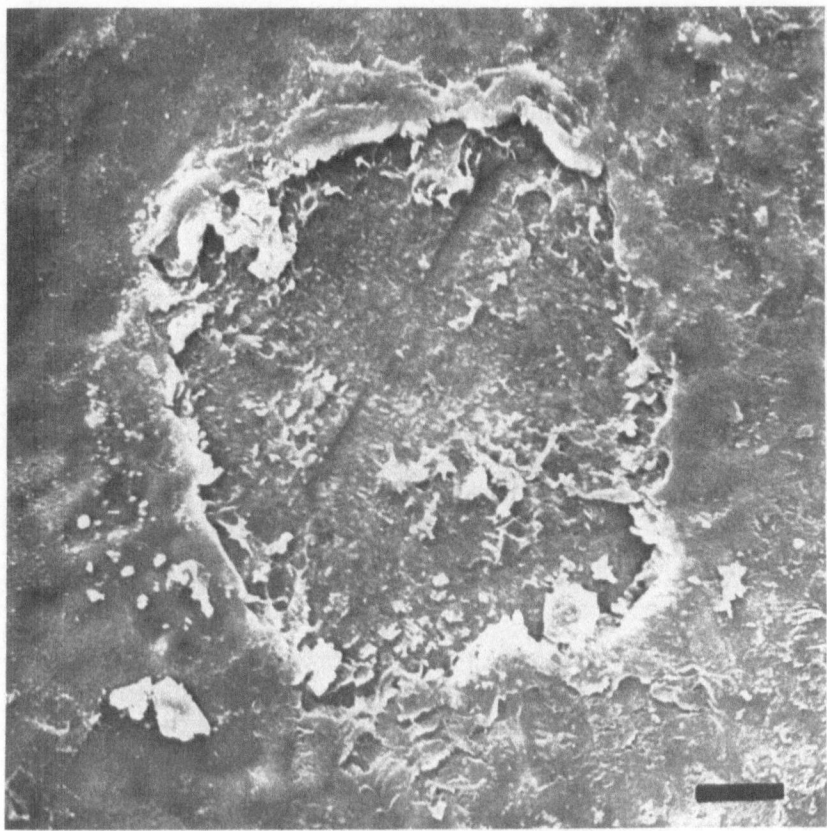

Fig. 58. Scanning electron microscopy of the corneal epithelium. Erosion of the superficial layers can be observed, as well as irregularity of the surface (× 128).

generated Bowman's membrane, lied against the base membrane. It was even possible to find these fibrils within the base membrane itself.

C. *Scanning electron microscopy*

By means of the scanning electron microscope, we studied the epithelial surface of a cornea affected by macular dystrophy:

1. This surface was very uneven, undulating and, in places, even anfractuous.

2. The nuclei protruded from the surface, but there were also cellular areas where they caused a rounded depression.

3. The intercellular spaces were mostly ill-defined. Some were much enlarged and crossed by cytoplasmic filiform bridges.

4. The cellular membrane displayed microvilli and microfolds of normal appearance.

5. In places, crateriform erosions having anfractuous edges and measuring on average 200 μm, were found (Fig. 58). They were produced at the expense of the most superficial layers or even of the whole thickness of the epithelium. The floors of these erosions showed numerous cell debris.

6. The epithelial surface showed polymorphic, grumous or filiform deposits.

II. CHANGES OF THE ENDOTHELIUM AND THE DESCEMET'S MEMBRANE.

All the corneas affected by macular dystrophy showed changes of the posterior limiting membranes (Figs. 59 to 61b). Histologically and histochemically, the lesions varied from one case to another.

1. In some cases, there were small endothelial vacuoles with some picnotic nuclei, the Descemet's membrane being apparently normal.

2. In other cases, there was a complete dystrophy of the posterior limiting membranes, with deterioration of the Descemet's membrane and storage of mucopolysaccharides in the endothelial cells.

a. *Clear-field microscopy of stained sections.*

1. *Haematoxylin-eosin* showed a Descemet's membrane either normal or of uneven thickness. In many cases, and above all the periphery, typical Hassall-Henle corpuscles could be seen. The nuclei of the endothelial cells, which appeared atrophic or globular, were mostly picnotic.

2. The *histochemical dyes* for the mucopolysaccharides (three cases) showed a storage of mucopolysaccharides in the corneal endothelium, consisting of granulations identical with those of the keratocytes. The Descemet's membrane could be duplicated, the two layers staining differently. In one of our cases, Alcian blue of pH 1 or 2.5 stained the anterior layer of the Descemet's membrane pink and the posterior layer blue-grey.

b. *At the polarisation microscope and the dark-field phase-contrast microscope*, these endothelial granulations of the mucopolysaccharides showed the same characteristics as in the keratocytes (Fig.s. 59, 60 and 61a and b).

c. *Electron microscopy*

We found changes of the posterior limiting membranes in all the three cases we examined (Fig. 62). In the least affected case, which had clinically normal posterior limiting membranes, we found an invasion of the anterior layers of the Descemet's membrane by vesicles measuring on an average 1.5 μm, as well as by small rounded granules of ribosomal appearance. The endothelial cells appeared to be normal.

In the most evolved case, various lesions could be observed:

a. The Descemet's membrane was invaded by numerous rounded or flat-

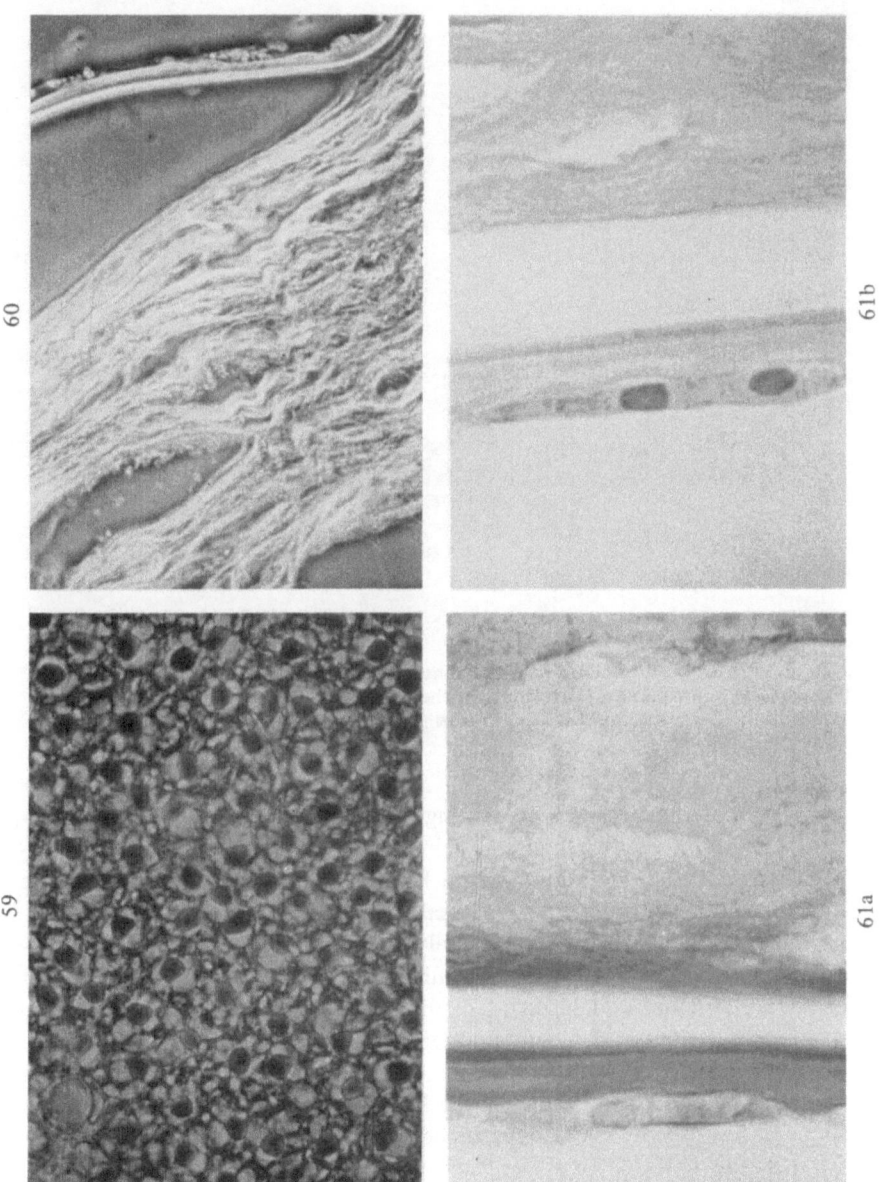

Fig. 59. Flat section of the endothelium. There are multiple cytoplasmic vacuoles and pycnotic nuclei (x 10 obj.).

Fig. 60. Fresh section of the posterior limiting membrane. Alterations of the Descemet's membrane. Cytoplasmic granulations in the endothelial cells (x 40 obj.).

Fig. 61. Storage of mucopolysaccharides in the endothelial cells. (a) Staining of Rinehart and Abul-Haj (x 40 obj.). (b) Alcian blue (pH 1) staining. The Descemet's membrane shows a double staining (grey in the posterior part and pink in the anterior part) (x 40 obj.).

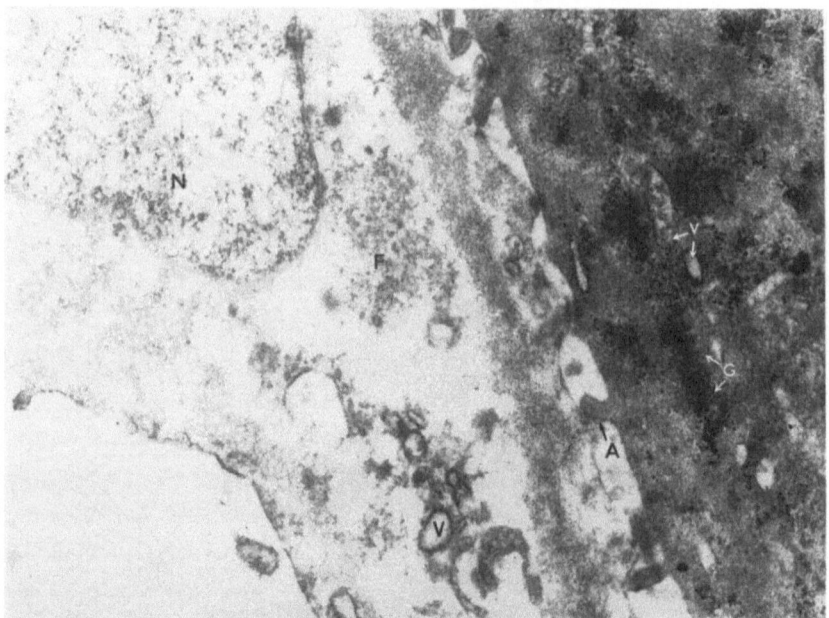

Fig. 62. Corneal endothelium with filamentous material (F). (N) nucleus). (v) vesicles. (G) granular material and (V) vesicles in the Descemet's membrane. (A) ties between the endothelium and the Descemet's membrane. Transmission electron microscopy (x 11 250).

tened membranous vesicles, measuring on an average 0.5 to 1 μm, and containing in some cases membrane debris or rounded, electron-dense inclusions, as well as granulations of the lysosomal type. The thickness of the membrane was not uniform, and Hassall-Henle corpuscles could be seen.

b. The endothelial cells were severely deteriorated. Their cytoplasm presented clear spaces filled with a granulo-filamentous material similar to that of the keratocytes and having a medium electron density. More electron-dense granulations and membrane debris could also be observed. In some cases, fascicles of tonofibrils surrounded clear cytoplasmic spaces. The ties between the endothelial cells and the Descemet's membrane were broken in some places, pseudovesicular spaces between the two structures being seen.

d. *Scanning electron microscopy*

The case that we observed was controlled histochemically. The posterior limiting membranes were severely deteriorated (Fig. 63).

1. *Endothelium.* The endothelial mosaic was irregular, because many cells were shrunken. The intercellular spaces were fairly large and crossed by the cytoplasmic ties linking one cell to another. In places, an endothelial erosion with uneven edges was observed. The endothelial cells surrounding the ero-

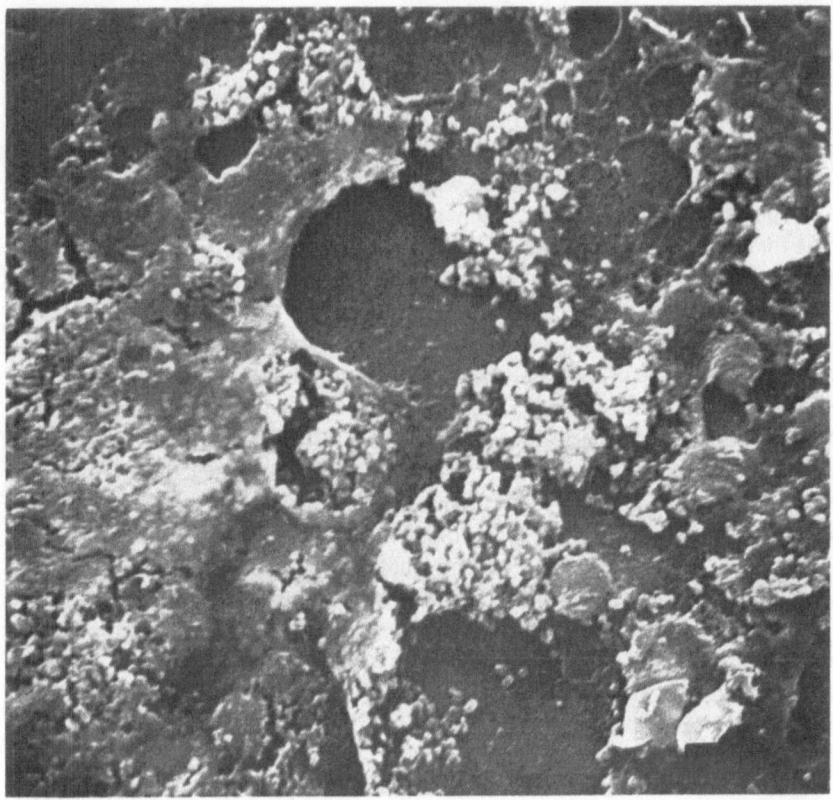

Fig. 63. Rupture of the endothelial mosaic and presence of many cellular debris. This photograph corresponds to the case of Fig. 44. Scanning transmission electron microscopy (x 1127).

sion was attached to the Descemet's membrane by fine pseudopodia. The erosion was filled with cell debris (Fig. 63). Irregular and granular deposits could be seen, apparently lying against the endothelial surface of the Descemet's membrane. They measured from 0.5 to 1 μm.

2. *Descemet's membrane.* This was lamellated and invaded by granular deposits identical with those of the posterior layer of the stroma. These granulations were more numerous in the anterior layers of the Descemet's membrane, where they were arranged in clots. In the posterior layers, they were smaller and more isolated.

DISCUSSION

All the changes observed in the epithelium were secondary to the lesions of the stroma. There was no pathognomonic change of the epithelium in macular dystrophy of the cornea. We cultivated epithelia obtained from corneas affected by macular dystrophy. After forty-eight hours, the culture showed completely normal cells, which indicated that when the epithelium is isolated from the pathological stroma, the epithelial cells become again normal, and, consequently, the lesions and deposits are secondary.

Concerning the endothelium, which is mesodermic and can store up mucopolysaccharides, the problem is more difficult. We believe, however, that the endothelial lesions are secondary. Indeed:

1. There are cases, wherein there is not yet an endothelial storage, whereas it manifestly exists in the keratocytes.

2. In cases with endothelial storage, the barrier constituted by the Descemet's membrane is broken, as it shows numerous lesions throughout its thickness. On the other hand, in the cases wherein the endothelium does not display any storage, the intermediate and posterior layers of the Descemet's membrane are undamaged. These facts are evident at the electron and scanning microscope. They argue in favour of an endothelial invasion originating from the stroma through the Descemet's membrane.

In view of the fact that the endothelial cells and the keratocytes have some characteristics in common (Hoof, 1948; Rohem, 1963), François et al. (1972c) do not exclude nevertheless that the changes might be primary in both types of cells.

3. It has not been demonstrated that the endothelial cells are capable of producing keratosulphate, which is the fundamental component of the stored material.

According to Jones et al. (1959), Morgan (1966), Lorenzetti et al. (1967), Thiel et al. (1971), Malbran (1972), Malbran et al. (1973), François et al. (1975a and b), the endothelial changes should rather be secondary.

CONCLUSION

From our studies, it may be concluded that in macular dystrophy of the cornea:

1. There exist various epithelial changes, which are nevertheless not specific. They are secondary to the large areas of subepithelial degeneration and may be accompanied by an invasion of macrophages. Intra- and intercellular epithelial oedema are also observed.

2. When the disease evolves in depth, the Descemet's membrane and the endothelium can be invaded. The Descemet's membrane is then affected before the endothelium. We never observed isolated endothelial lesions. The invasion of the posterior limiting membranes is evident at the scanning microscope.

3. The mucopolysaccharide granules found in the cytoplasm of the endothelial cells are identical with those stored by the keratocytes.

CHAPTER XI

HISTOCHEMICAL AND MICROSCOPICAL STUDY OF CORNEAL CULTURES FROM MACULAR DYSTROPHY

PERSONAL OBSERVATIONS

We were the first to cultivate keratocytes from macular dystrophy of the cornea.

I. DEVELOPMENT OF THE CULTURES

Fourty-eight hours after the implantation cell movements could be observed. A meshwork of cells with dark granulations developed in the thickness of the implanted stroma.

After seventy-two hours, the first cells appeared outside the specimen. They formed an irregular meshwork layered in one or more planes.

Between the fifth and the eighth day, the cells spread out farther over the monolayer taking rounded, curved or rectilinear shapes. They showed numerous vacuoles. Debris and extracellular granulations could be seen.

The cell mortality rate was very high. Although cell divisions were numerous, the growth rate of the cultures during the logarithmic phase was not high.

After the twentieth day, cytolytic phenomena were observed in all the flasks. Numerous debris adhered to the plasma clot or floated in the medium.

Subcultures grew readily, but after twenty-four hours, cytolytic phenomena were already seen.

In one case, all the culture flasks showed lytic phenomena by the third month, causing the death of all the cells. The subcultures grew with more difficulty. However, it was possible to obtain enough cells by reimplanting the specimens, which grew as if they were in a primoculture.

In another case, the cultures were negative, the fragments detaching from the glass surface after a few hours. An histological examination of the implantation tissue showed the absence of viable cells. Numerous keratocytes were destroyed. The reactions for acid phosphatase were strongly positive at the level of the remaining cell fragments, which confirmed the cellular autolysis.

139

II. EXAMINATION OF THE IMPLANTATION SPECIMEN

After forty-eight hours and fifteen days of implantation, some fragments had not grown, whereas others had produced a large number of keratocytes. There were also specimens with apparently living keratocytes, but also some which showed no sign of growth.

III. MICROSCOPY

A. *Implanted fragment*

a. At the *phase-contrast microscope*, the unstained sections showed very numerous keratocytes, which migrated toward the periphery of the specimen. They were characterised by intracytoplasmic storage granules. Many of them burst during their movement toward the periphery. A deposit of more or less disseminated granules without nuclei could then be seen.

Areas of collagenous lysis could be observed, and, in some cases, areolar areas, above all around the cells in progression. These areas were stained pink by PAS, saffron being negative. The Van Gieson and Wilder methods stained them only slightly.

b. The *histochemical study at the clear-field microscope* showed that the granules had the same characteristics as on the histological sections. After the rupture of the cells, they formed a deposit identical with that found between the corneal lamellae 'in situ' (Fig. 66). The only remarkable fact was the presence of RNA, demonstrated by the acridine-orange staining, which gave a positive fluorescence, partially negatived by ribonuclease. On the edges of the specimen, numerous storage granules could be found, forming a band of 20 to 40 μm.

c. At the *polarisation microscope*, the birefringence was absent in extensive areas. There remained, nevertheless, a certain number of tortuous collagen fascicles, which appeared to be normal, both in fresh sections and after staining (Fig. 65).

d. At the *dark-field microscope*, extensive areas of deteriorated collagen were observed. The lytic areas consisted of innumerable polychromic spots after staining by the Van Gieson or Wilder method. There remained nevertheless some fascicles of normal appearance.

B. *Keratocytes in monolayer*

a. *Phase-contrast microscopy of fresh monolayers.* The primocultures and the subcultures displayed similar characteristics, two of which were obvious

140

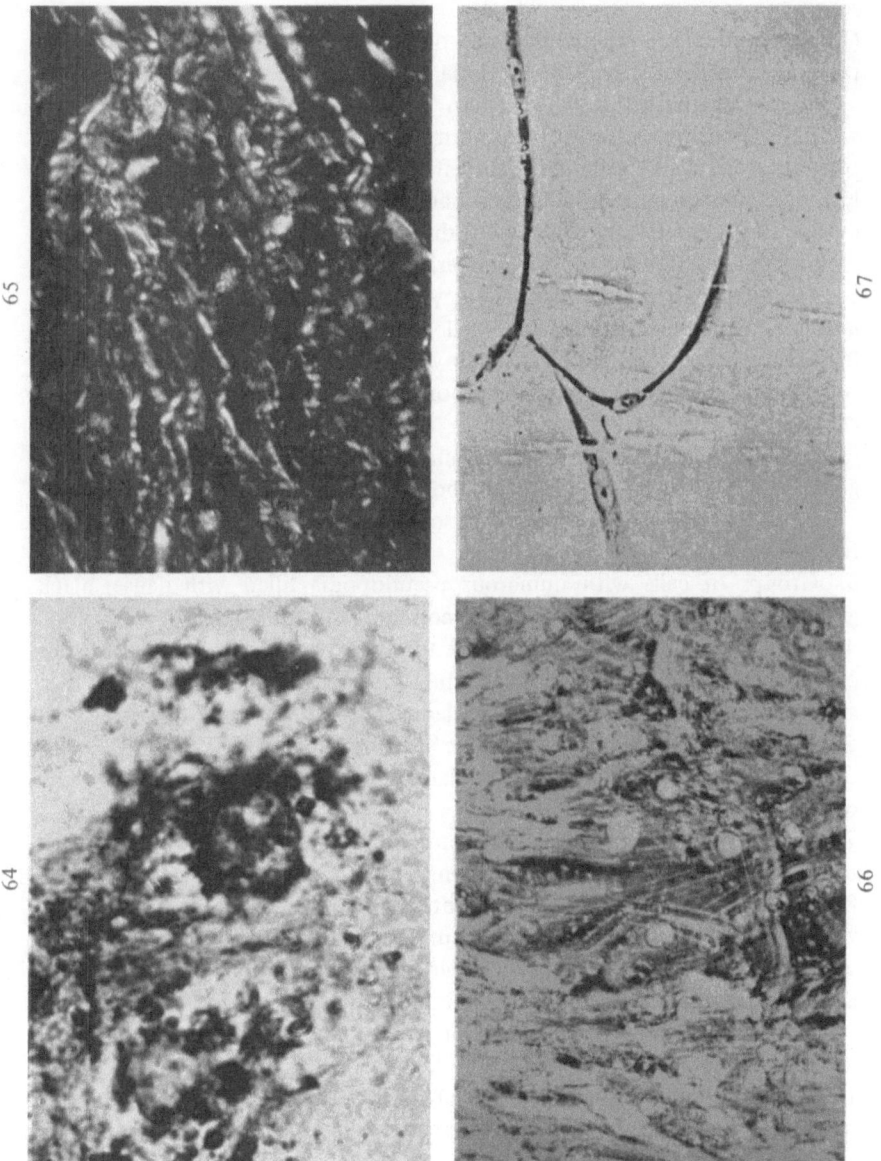

Fig. 64. Development of two keratocytes in the specimen. Osmophilous granulations (brown). Staining with Alcian blue after fixation with osmic acid (x 100 obj.).

Fig. 65. Development of keratocytes in the specimen. Mucopolysaccharidic granulations with blue birefringence. The collagen has a brown birefringence. Rinehart and Abul-Haj (x 20 obj.).

Fig. 66. Monolayer culture. Disorganised growth of the cells and death of numerous elements (x 20 obj.).

Fig. 67. Monolayer culture. Keratocytes with atrophied cytoplasm completely filled with granules (x 20 obj.).

141

(Figs. 66 and 67): (i) the presence of numerous cell debris, and (ii) the presence of cells of very different dimensions.

At low magnification, the pattern of the cells was irregular, compared with the arciform pattern of the normal keratocytes. At higher magnification, the cells were rather different one from another. They had, nevertheless, one characteristic in common, namely the presence of very numerous cytoplasmic granulations of different dimensions and optical densities.

We shall describe the most characteristic cells:

1. Rounded cells, which displayed a cytoplasm filled with small grey granulations. At the periphery of these cells, clots of black granules were found, in some cases surrounded by a white vacuolar area. They contained numerous tonofibrils. Their nuclei were normal and contained one or two nucleoli.

2. Triangular cells with three primary pseudopodia, containing dense granules of 0.5 to 1 μm. The cell bodies contained grey granulations of 1 μm, surrounded by paler zones. In some cases these granulations took the form of small rods.

3. Groups of cells with numerous pseudopodia filled with dense, black granulations and converging toward a common centre.

4. Oval cells with four to six very thin pseudopodia at each pole. The cytoplasm was filled with grey granulations of 0.5 μm. The nucleus was slightly eccentric and contained a nucleolus.

5. Cells similar to the preceding cells, but rounded.

6. Racket-shaped cells with denser black granulations in the primary pseudopodium.

7. Cells with three pseudopodia, containing black granulations, separated by clearer spaces. Each nucleus contained three nucleoli.

8. Elongated or fusiform cells, containing grey granulations and white vacuoles which in many cases surrounded the granules. The nucleus was oval. Its longest axis was perpendicular to the longest axis of the cell. This arrangement has never been observed in normal cells.

9. Triangular cells containing grey or black granulations and vacuoles. The nucleus was very small and pressed back against the cell membrane.

10. Fusiform cells, wherein the nucleus divided the cytoplasm into two parts, one being occupied by granulations and the other by a black mass consisting of grouped granules and surrounded by an apparently empty white vacuolar space.

11. Cells similar to the preceding cells, except that the agglomerated granules have been eliminated. There remained the nucleus, which occupied one pole of the cell, and the cytoplasm, which contained grey granules.

12. Cells having an abundant cytoplasm, filled with grey or black granulations. They contained two central nuclei, each of which containing one nucleolus.

142

13. Atrophic cells, the cytoplasm of which was thin and elongated, attaining more than 50 μm. It was completely filled with black granulations. The nucleus was small and contained one or two nucleoli.

14. Cells whose bodies contained grey granulations of 0.5 μm and extended up to 30 μm or more in order to reach other cell bodies. These cytoplasmic bridges contained very dense black granulations.

15. In some cases, two or three cells were grouped. Their nuclei were displaced toward the periphery. A part of the cytoplasm was vacuolised and partitioned, containing debris, whereas another part contained grey granulations.

16. Some cells had long fine pseudopodia, which displayed rounded enlargements filled with black granules.

Table 11. Histochemistry of the keratocytes of macular dystrophy of the cornea in tissue culture.

Methods	Granules	Large vacuoles	Large empty vacuoles
Colloidal iron	+	+	−
Alcian blue, pH 1	+	+	−
Alcian blue, pH 2.5	+	+	−
Metachromatic curve	Metachromasia values	at all pH	unstained
Direct Schiff	−	−	−
PAS (5 min. oxidation with periodic acid)	+	+	−
PAS (15 min. oxidation with periodic acid)	+	+	−
Oil Red "0"	−	−	+
Reticulin	−	+ in some vacuoles	−

Methods		Granules	Large vacuoles	Large empty vacuoles	Nucleus
Acridine Orange	RNA red fluorescence	The cytoplasm shows an irregular distribution of RNA around the vacuoles			+
	DNA green fluorescence	−	+ in some cases	−	+ in the nucleoli
Acid phosphatase		+	+	−	
Hyaluronidase test		−	−		
Birefringence (polarisation microscopy)		Birefingence of the membranes, but not of the vacuoles			absent

−Negative   +Weakly positive   [   ]   Method inapplicable

17. Groups of cells in the course of lysis could be seen. Black granules, surrounded by white vacuolar spaces, were found outside the cells. Membrane debris and tonofibrils were still attached to the monolayer, but it was no longer possible to distinguish nuclei.

b. *Histochemical study (Table XI).*

1. *Haemotoxylin-eosin staining.* The cytoplasmic matrix was eosinophil and stained pale pink. The vacuoles and the granulations were not stained. The nucleus was strongly basophil.

2. *Staining of the reticulin according to Wilder (Fig. 68).* This was positive in some peripheral areas and in some granulations. It was negative in the large vacuoles and in most of the granules.

3. *Staining by Van Gieson's method.* It was weakly positive, above all at the periphery, although it was negative in the granulations and the large cytoplasmic vacuoles.

4. *Staining with colloidal iron according to Rinehart and Abul-Haj.* It was positive, although the staining intensity was not very high, because of the thinness of the culture cells. It was positive both in the granules, as well as in the large vacuoles, which were not black at the phase-contrast microscope. Some large vacuoles, however, remained negative.

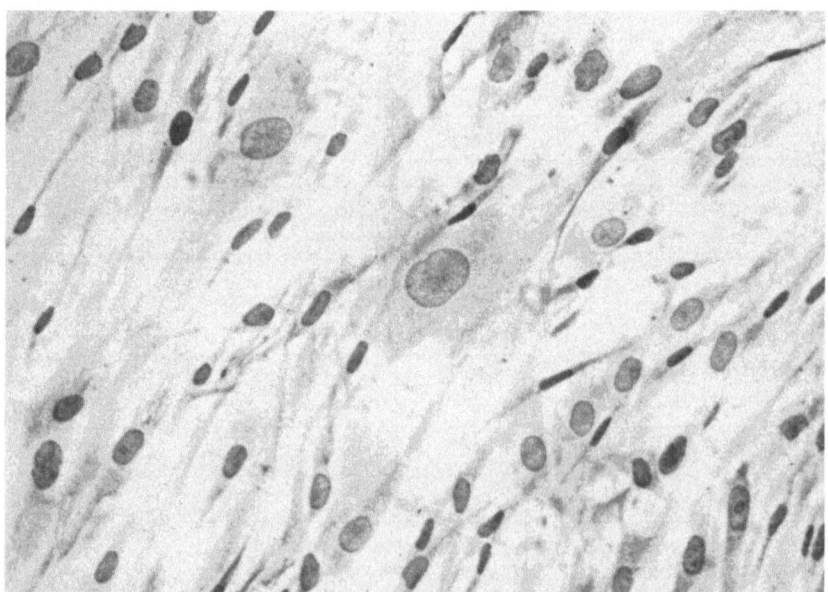

Fig. 68. Monolayer culture. Reticulin granulations (brown) in the cytoplasm. Wilder's method (x 20 obj.).

5. *Alcian blue* both at pH 1 and pH 2.5 was positive for the structures, which were positive for colloidal iron. The calcium-chloride neutralisation test gave results identical with those observed in the keratocytes affected by macular dystrophy 'in situ', that is to say, than in order to neutralise the staining for pH 1 Alcian blue, it was necessary to treat the sections beforehand with a magnesium chloride solution, the concentration of which was at least 1.3 M.

6. *Metachromatic curve for toluidine blue.* The material stored in the large vacuoles and in most of the granules was metachromatic. The metachromasia might be either type β or type γ. In the nucleolus, there were irregularly distributed areas of α or β metachromasia. The periphery of the nucleolus was rather orthochromatic.

7. The *direct Schiff reaction* was negative and no free aldehyde groups could be detected by this method.

8. *Staining with periodic acid Schiff (PAS) (Fig. 69).* The cytoplasmic matrix was slightly positive. It became so only after fifteen minutes of oxidation by periodic acid. On the other hand, most of the granules and large vacuoles were positive after five minutes of oxidation. There were, however, some apparently empty vacuoles which were not stained. The nuclei were not stained.

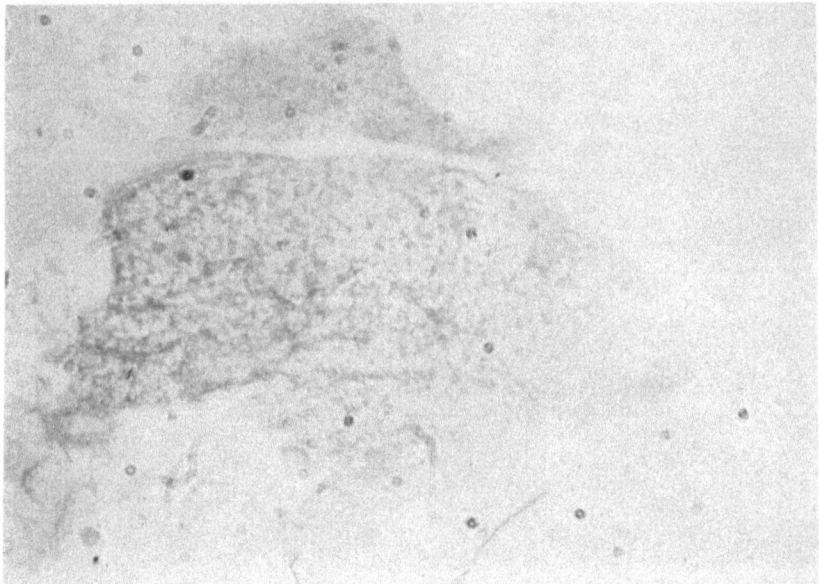

Fig. 69. Monolayer culture. Positive granulations in the cytoplasm. PAS with oxidation during five minutes (x 50 obj.).

9. *Staining for lipids.* Numerous vacuoles were positive for Oil Red 'O', Sudan III and Sudan black, whereas the cytoplasmic granulations were negative. The Schultze reaction for cholesterol was negative in the vacuoles.

10. *Acridine orange staining according to Mortelmans and Sebruyns* (Fig. 70). The cytoplasm showed large negative vacuolar spaces, surrounded by cytoplasm partly positive for RNA. However, the perivacuolar positivity was irregular, the orange-red fluorescence varying from one vacuole to another, or even within one and the same vacuole. These large vacuolar spaces represented dilated ergastoplasmic cisterns. In addition, medium or small vacuoles were observed, which were also negative and surrounded by an irregular orange-red fluorescence.

In the nucleus, the distribution of the green DNA fluorescence could be normal. It was more irregular when the nucleus was distorted. The nucleus could also be positive for RNA, the fluorescence varying from orange-yellow to red.

At the phase-contrast microscope, the morphological changes of the cytoplasm and the nucleus were still more evident after staining with acridine orange.

11. *Ribonuclease test.* The cells treated beforehand by ribonuclease no longer displayed an orange-red fluorescence of the cytoplasm and nucleoli, which confirmed the presence of RNA.

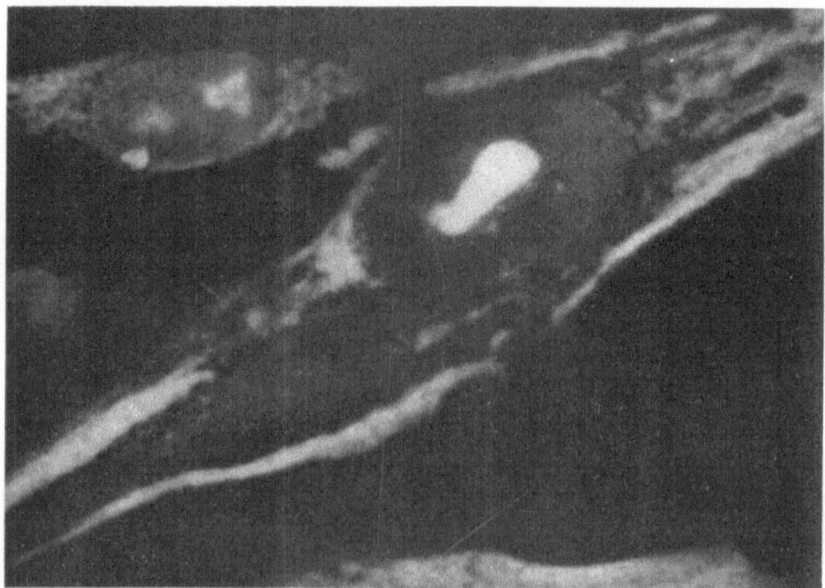

Fig. 70. Monolayer culture. Mortelmans and Sebruyns method. RNA (red) surrounds large cisterns (black). Nucleoli containing RNA (orange). Fluorescence microscopy (× 50 obj.).

12. *Hyaluronidase test.* Treatment with bovine testicular hyaluronidase did not inhibit the staining by colloidal iron, pH 1 to pH 2.5 Alcian blue, toluidine blue or PAS.

13. *The Takeuchi and Tanoue staining for acid phosphatase* was positive for most of the granulations and the large vacuoles (Fig. 71).

c. *Polarisation microscopy* (Fig. 72). Birefringence was observed throughout the cytoplasm. Numerous membranous folds and certain granules were also birefringent. All the birefringent structures disappeared after treatment of the cells by organic solvents.

It must be stressed that, in most of the granules and vacuoles, there was no birefringence. When the cells were stained with Alcian blue or PAS, the few granules and vacuoles, which were birefringent before staining, were no longer so, notwithstanding that the cells had not been treated with organic solvents.

d. *Phase-contrast microscopy of the histochemically stained monolayers* merely confirmed the observations at the clear-field microscope. In the layers stained with Fast Red, abnormal mitoses could be observed. The study of the metaphases showed, indeed, between 20 and 30% of polyploid mitoses.

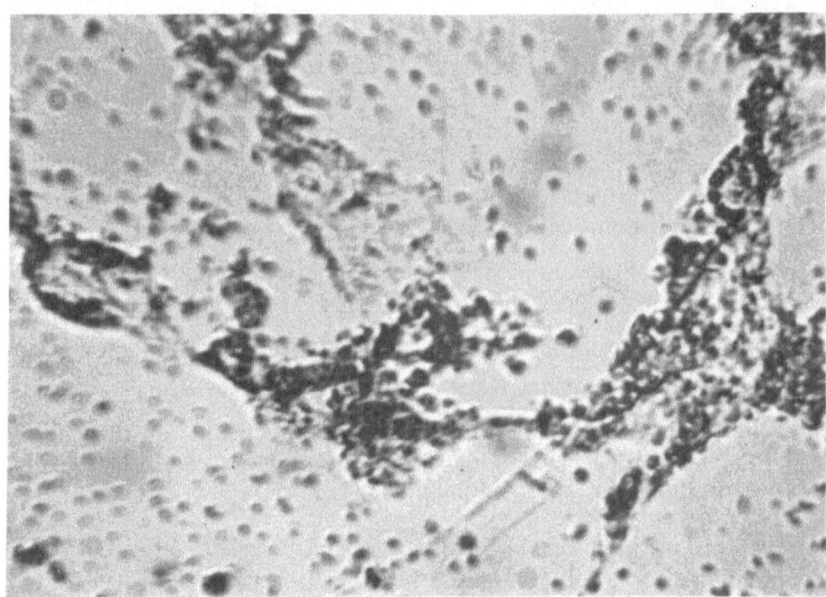

Fig. 71. Monolayer culture. Positive granulations in the cytoplasm. Acid phosphatase according to Takeuchi and Tanoue (x 25 obj.).

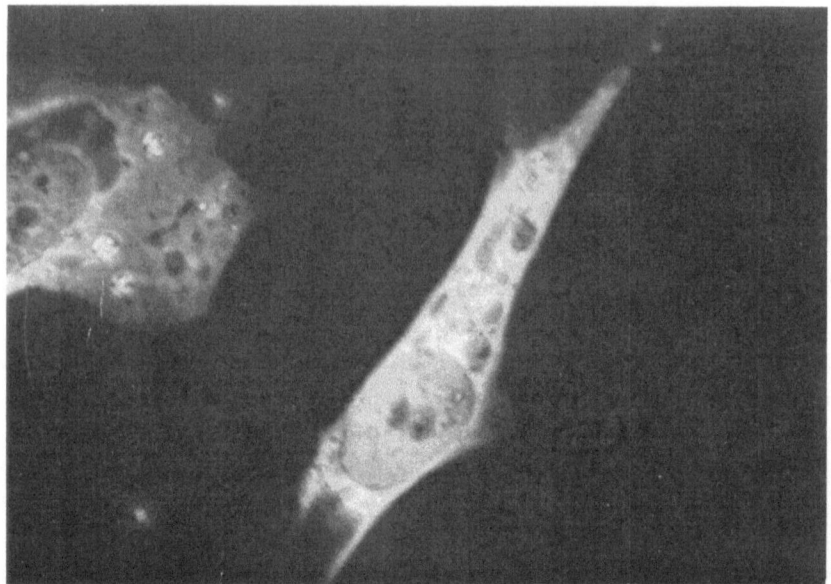

Fig. 72. Monolayer culture. Fresh cells. A cytoplasmic birefringence and vacuolar spaces are observed. Polarisation microscopy (× 50 obj.).

e. *Dark-field microscopy of the histochemically stained monolayers.*

1. *Periodic-acid Schiff (PAS).* In the cytoplasm, small dots of bright-red staining, measuring 0.1 μm, were seen. In addition, very bright granules of about 1 μm were found, their staining varying from red to golden yellow, as well as large, optically empty vacuolar spaces surrounded by small or medium granulations, large vacuolar spaces occupied by bright, red or yellow dots, and large, bright, silver-white vacuoles measuring more than 2 μm. The cytoplasm was apparently partitioned by fine, bright brownish lines, which were probably of membranous origin.

2. *Alcian blue.* Most of the small or medium granulations were stained blue-green. At pH 2.5, the staining was bluer and at pH 1, greener.

3. *Colloidal iron according to Rinehart and Abul-Haj* stained the small and medium granulations green.

4. *Staining of the reticulin according to Wilder.* At the places where at the clear field microscope the staining was positive, innumerable bright golden dots were found at the dark-field microscope.

5. *The Takeuchi and Tanoue staining for acid phosphatase* showed bright silverish punctiform deposits in the very small elements, which were not visible at the clear-field microscope.

148

DISCUSSION

It is possible to cultivate keratocytes obtained from a macular dystrophy of the cornea. It is, nevertheless, indispensable to implant the corneal specimen not more than two hours after its removal. The cellular autolysis develops, indeed, very rapidly and inhibits the growth of the culture. In the case of primocultures, the keratocytes develop first inside and later outside the specimen. The appearance of the cells is very variable.

The development of the pathological keratocytes produces areas of lysis in the stroma of the specimen, where the reactions for acid phosphatase, indicative of lysosomal activity, are highly positive.

During their migration within the specimen, numerous keratocytes burst, liberating cytoplasmic granulations highly positive for stainings of mucopolysaccharides and acid phosphatase. At that level, the collagen is destroyed, the first sign of its deterioration being the loss of birefringence.

The subcultures develop readily when the cultures are fresh, but with great difficulty after the fourth month. Nevertheless, phenomena of cellular lysis are very soon observed, together with the formation of numerous debris, which remain adhering to the slide or float in the culture medium.

Fresh monolayers show phenomena of very intense cytolysis and very pronounced cellular anisomorphism.

Various cytoplasmic inclusions are found:
1. Very small granulations of 0.1 μm, visible only at the dark-field microscope. These granulations are positive for the stainings of mucopolysaccharides and acid phosphatase.
2. Granules measuring 0.5 to 1 μm, also positive for mucopolysaccharides. Most of them are also positive for acid phosphatase.
3. Vacuoles measuring about 2 μm, positive for mucopolysaccharides and lipids, which might be due to the lipopolysaccharide matrix of the lysosomes. Many of the vacuoles, however, do not stain and are optically empty at the dark-field microscope.
4. Vacuoles, which merge to form large vacuolar spaces, are clearly visible after staining with acridine orange, because they are delimited by the red fluorescence of the RNA. Smaller granulations are in many cases arranged around the vacuoles.

The membranes, which are clearly visible at the polarisation microscope, are highly developed.

The birefringent lipid structures disappear after treatment with organic solvents.

There are areas of collagen neoformation, demonstrated by Wilder's method and the Van Gieson staining.

In many cases the nuclei of the keratocytes are abnormal and displaced toward the periphery of the cell. The presence of 20 to 30% of polyploid nuclei indicates a genetic deterioration in the growth of the cultures. Indeed, the number of polyploid mitoses does not exceed 2% in cultures of normal keratocytes.

The histochemical study *in vivo* and the examination at the phase-contrast microscope of both the implanted specimen and the monolayers, show the pathological process of macular dystrophy of the cornea. The most important fact is that the lesions of the corneal stroma are due to cytolytic phenomena accompanied by the liberation of lysosomal enzymes, which digest the neighbouring tissues. All these lesions are, indeed, positive for acid phosphatase.

In another study, we proposed a pathogenesis for macular dystrophy of the cornea (François and Victoria-Troncoso, 1975) (see chapter XVI). The tissue culture provides us with further proofs in favour of our theory.

CONCLUSIONS

1. The tissue culture of macular dystrophy of the cornea makes it possible to observe the accelerated evolution of the dystrophy and the formation of further lesions of the corneal stroma due to the developing keratocytes. These lesions are thus secondary to the alteration of the keratocytes.

2. The disease consists in the storage of keratosulphate, which can be followed up to the death of the cell. The observations made on tissue cultures correspond to those made on biopsies and demonstrate indisputably the *primary involvement of the keratocytes*, as well as the secondary involvement of the neighbouring structures.

3. The mortality rate of the cells is very high and their span of life is very short. On the other hand, their growth is accelerated. If the same phenomena occur *'in situ'*, the disease must be accompanied by a hyperproduction of cells and of corneal mucopolysaccharides.

4. The activity of the lysosomes is important, because granules are found in the corneal specimen after rupture of the cells. The lysosomal origin of these granules is demonstrated by the positive staining for acid phosphatase.

5. Tissue culture made it possible to observe, for the first time, the behaviour *in vivo* of pathological keratocytes, showing an inborn error of the metabolism of keratosulphate.

6. The culture of keratocytes from macular dystrophy will make possible enzymological studies *in vivo* as well as therapeutical research.

CHAPTER XII

TRANSMISSION ELECTRON MICROSCOPY OF CULTURES OF THE CORNEAL STROMA IN MACULAR DYSTROPHY

PERSONAL OBSERVATIONS

We examined a certain number of monolayers at the electron microscope, in order to investigate the internal cell structure and the stored material.

The study of the implantation specimen revealed the same lesions as seen in the anatomical pieces. The keratocytes developed both inside and outside the specimen. The intracytoplasmic appearance was similar in the two cases we could examine (Fig. 73). In the vicinity of the cells, the specimen displayed, in addition, areas of lysis. The cells themselves were vacuolated and contained numerous inclusions. The cellular membrane was in many cases ruptured, allowing the organelles to leave the cell.

We found the following cytoplasmic cell structures (Figs. 73 and 74):

1. Rounded particles of 0.1 μm close to the Golgi's apparatus. Their matrix was of the lysosomal type. They had a velvety appearance and in some cases displayed fine white spaces. Their electron density was moderate.

2. Granulations of the lysosomal type, denser in some places.

3. Granulations of the lysosomal type, of velvety appearance, some parts of them showing a very high electron density.

4. Larger elements exceeding 1 μm and containing the same velvety material.

5. White vacuoles, apparently empty or containing only membranous debris.

6. Large vacuoles measuring more than 1 μm, containing a material arranged in dark parallel membranes alternating with clear bands. The periodicity of this material was 120 Å.

7. Vesicles containing other, smaller vesicles, whose electron density was variable (multivesicular bodies).

8. Vesicles of various dimensions, but exceeding mostly 1 μm, containing a granulo-filamentous material in loose meshes.

9. Granulations of the lysosomal type, containing a granular material.

10. Grouped granulations of the lysosomal type, containing a material, whose density varied from one granulation to another.

11. Granules of the lysosomal type containing a material of low electron density, although there were spots of high electron density. Some parts of the membrane surrounding them showed also in some cases high electron density.

12. Particles of the lysosomal type, with velvety or granular contents and showing partitioned white spaces of various dimensions. In some cases these lysosomes contained spots of very high electron density.

13. The intralysosomal material was sometimes shrunken and detached from the membrane.

14. Large granules of the lysosomal type filled with a granular material, including some denser spots. Centrally or eccentrally, there was a single rounded, very electron-dense body. Granules of this type were frequently seen.

15. Vesicles whose central part was empty and in which a granular material was seen, lying against the surrounding membrane.

16. Two vesicles arranged concentrically, the one inside the other. The inner vesicle contained granular material. The space between the inner and outer membranes appeared to be empty.

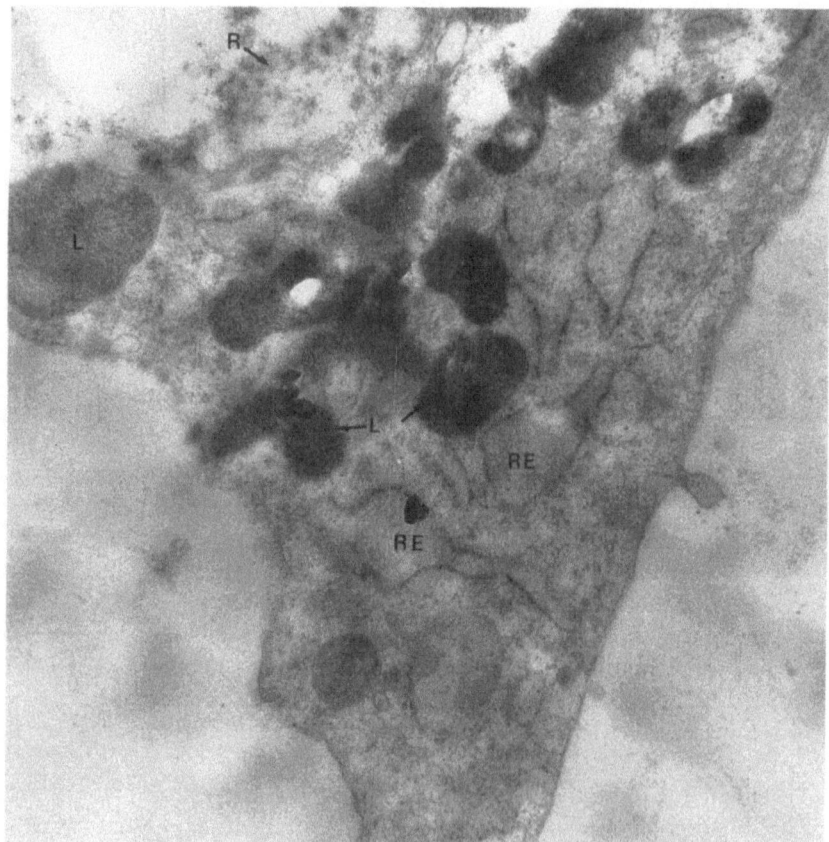

Fig. 73. Cytoplasm of a keratocyte outside the specimen. (L) lysosome (F) long spacing fibres. (RE) endoplasmic reticulum (x 5500).

17. Multivesicular bodies, which displayed loose filamentous meshes as well as two or three other vesicles of higher electron density.

18. In some cases, merging vesicles and granules of the lysosomal type, the material passing from one to the other.

All these particles were not necessarily intracellular. It happened that the cell bursts, particles being then found inside the specimen or adhering to the monolayer.

In many cases, very different granulations were grouped in a rolled-up 'ball' of granulo-filamentous material.

19. We can still find the accumulation of the following material in the keratocytes or outside the cells in the stroma of the specimen:

a. A characteristic structure consisted of large *cytoplasmic spaces containing a collagen material*, which displayed a periodicity of 2800 Å, whereas the adult collagen has a periodicity of 680 Å. These fibres, called 'long spacing fibres' (LSF), were found in the Descemet's membrane at the level of the Hassall-Henle corpuscles (Fig. 73).

b. A finely granular material without membranous envelope.

c. A filamentous material forming loose meshes.

d. A material of velvety appearance.

e. A material consisting of parallel electron-dense sheets, having a periodicity of 120 Å. This material was identical with that seen in anatomical pieces.

20. The *endoplasmic reticulum* was dilated. It might be granular and contain numerous ribosomes. The ergastoplasmic cisterns could be apparently empty or contain one of the materials already described. The ergastoplasmic membrane, which partially enveloped the cistern, fused with numerous lysosomes, which spilt their contents into the ergastoplasmic space.

21. The *Golgi's apparatus* was hypertrophic. It displayed a very large number of vacuoles and numerous parallel cisterns, which were more developed than in normal cultivated keratocytes. In addition, small granules of the lysosomal type with variable contents were found. In some of the cells, two or three apparently independent Golgi's apparatus could be observed.

22. The *mitochondria* were either normal or deteriorated. In the latter case, a vacuolisation, as well as concentric or partitioning membranes could be observed. The partitioning membranes united irregularly various points of the inner mitochondrial membrane, without forming real crests. In many cases the mitochondria were dilated at the expense of the mitochondrial space, which separated the outer and inner membranes.

23. The nucleolus was well developed. It contained granules, precursors of ribosomes, and filaments, precursors of granules. They were distributed in the trabecular structures known as nucleolonemas, which were separated by pale rounded spaces. We have never observed a segregation of the granular and filamentous parts, which mixed up.

The chromatin was perinucleolar and did not form intranuclear clumps.

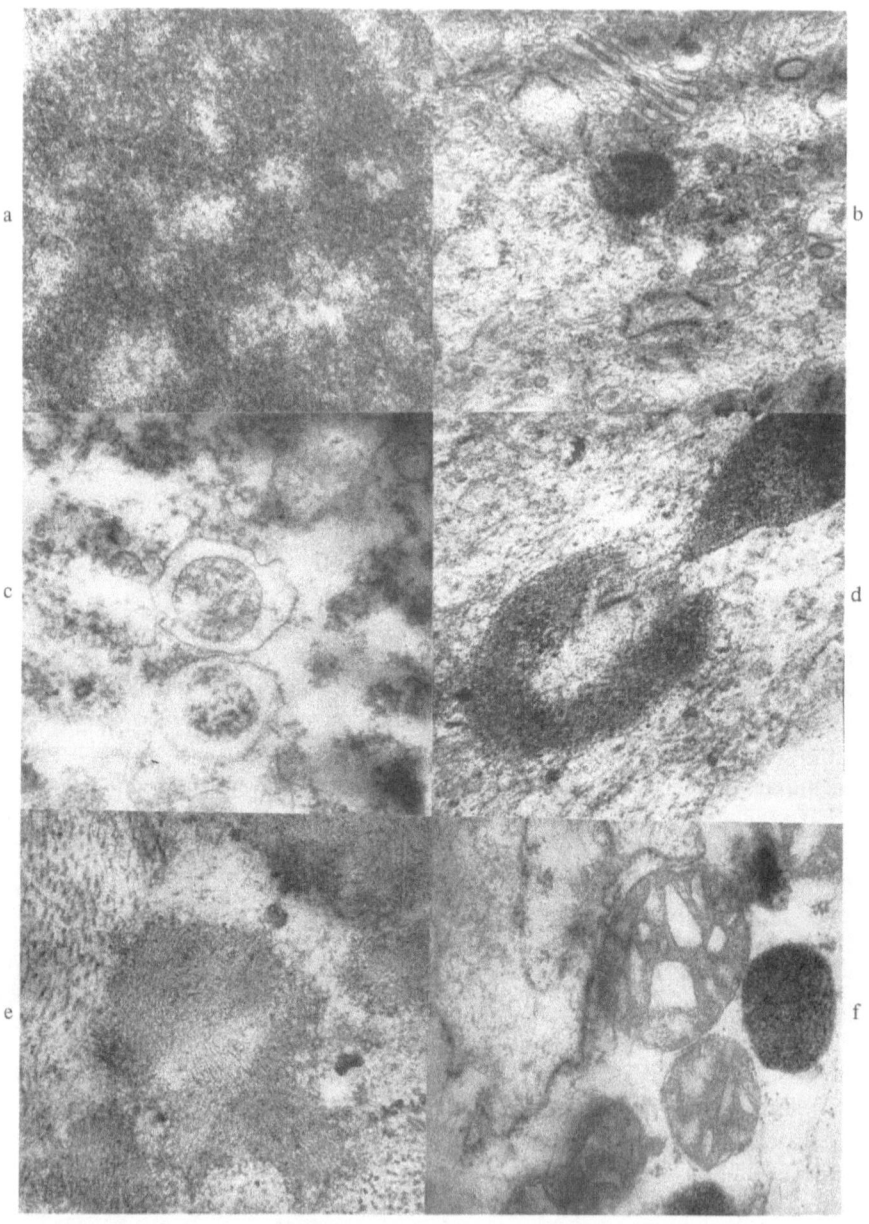

Fig. 74. Organelles of pathological keratocytes in tissue culture: (a) nucleoli. The nucleolonemas (grey) surround clear spaces (× 45 000). (b) Golgi's apparatus and a lysosome (× 17 500). (c) Multivesicular bodies (× 15 000). (d) Fusion of two lysosomes (× 45 000). (e) Periodic material in the specimen (× 17 500). (f) Two pathological mitochondria and two lysosomes (× 26 500).

154

The nucleolus itself was normal; it appeared to be very active, demonstrating an intensive production of the precursors of ribosomes and a high activity of cell biosynthesis.

DISCUSSION

The transmission electron microscope shows that numerous keratocytes develop during the course of corneal cell cultures obtained from macular dystrophy, and that they display essentially the same changes as pathological keratocytes *in situ*. There are numerous particles of variable dimensions. They are surrounded by membranes and show lysosomal characteristics.

An interesting lesion, that we have not observed *in situ*, consists of long spacing fibres, which indicate the precipitation of tropocollagen molecules and which have a periodicity of 2800 Å. This precipitation depends upon the nature of the neighbouring mucopolysaccharides. Normally, their molecules are precipitated in order to overlap the neighbouring molecules by a quarter of their length, producing fibrils whose periodicity is a quarter of the overall length of the molecule ($2800 \div 4 \approx 680$ Å).

CONCLUSIONS

The electron microscopy of cultures of macular dystrophy of the corneal shows:
1. Deteriorations in the vacuolar system. There are particles of different types, many of which resemble those observed *in situ*.
2. Morphological changes of the mitochondria.
3. Long spacing fibres in the dilated intracytoplasmic spaces.
4. Dilated endoplasmic reticulum.
5. Numerous degenerating cells.
6. Normal nuclei and nucleoli.

CHAPTER XIII

SCANNING ELECTRON MICROSCOPY OF THE CULTURES OF MACULAR DYSTROPHY OF THE CORNEA

PERSONAL OBSERVATIONS

We examined at the scanning electron microscope a number of monolayers obtained from two cases of macular dystrophy of the cornea, prepared according to the technique of François et al. (1973).

Comparative study of normal keratocytes and keratocytes affected by macular dystrophy (Figs. 75 and 76)

When normal keratocytes were compared with those of macular dystrophy, the differences were obvious.

1. The cellular surface was very anfractuous. It showed ridges and troughs, giving the impression that the cell was depressed or collapsed.

2. There were pseudopodia of only the first order, their surfaces being also very anfractuous.

3. Groups of granules covered by a membrane were found, adhering perfectly to the specimen holder. These granules were completely separated from the body of the cell, which was a few microns away. These granules showed excrescences in a glove shape.

4. The cells were of various dimensions and shapes. Smaller elements of atrophic appearance could be found. In some cases, the cell was completely spread out on the specimen holder. The nucleus and the nucleolus then protruded from the surface and the cell membrane was crossed by raised tonofibrils, which were put under tension in the underlying cytoplasm.

As we mentioned, normal keratocytes show pseudopodia of the first order (large pseudopodia prolonging the cell body), pseudopodia of the second order (pseudopodia protruding from first-order pseudopodia) and pseudopodia of the third order (multiple, fine pseudopodia leaving second-order pseudopodia). These pseudopodia were attached to the monolayer. The keratocytes of macular dystrophy of the cornea, on the contrary, had only first-order pseudopodia.

Whereas the surface of the cell bodies of normal keratocytes is smooth at the scanning microscope, that of the cells from macular dystrophy was irregular and anfractuous. Parts of the cytoplasm broke away from the cell body during the movements of the keratocytes. This phenomenon explains the presence in the stroma of isolated elements whose cellular origin was not demonstrated. The scanning microscope provides the proof, since it showed only cells developing outside the specimen.

The cellular anisomorphism and the atrophic cells, which were seen in macular dystrophy of the cornea, but never in a normal cornea, might also be observed at the phase-contrast microscope. However, alongside abnormal cells, some cells of normal appearance could also be found.

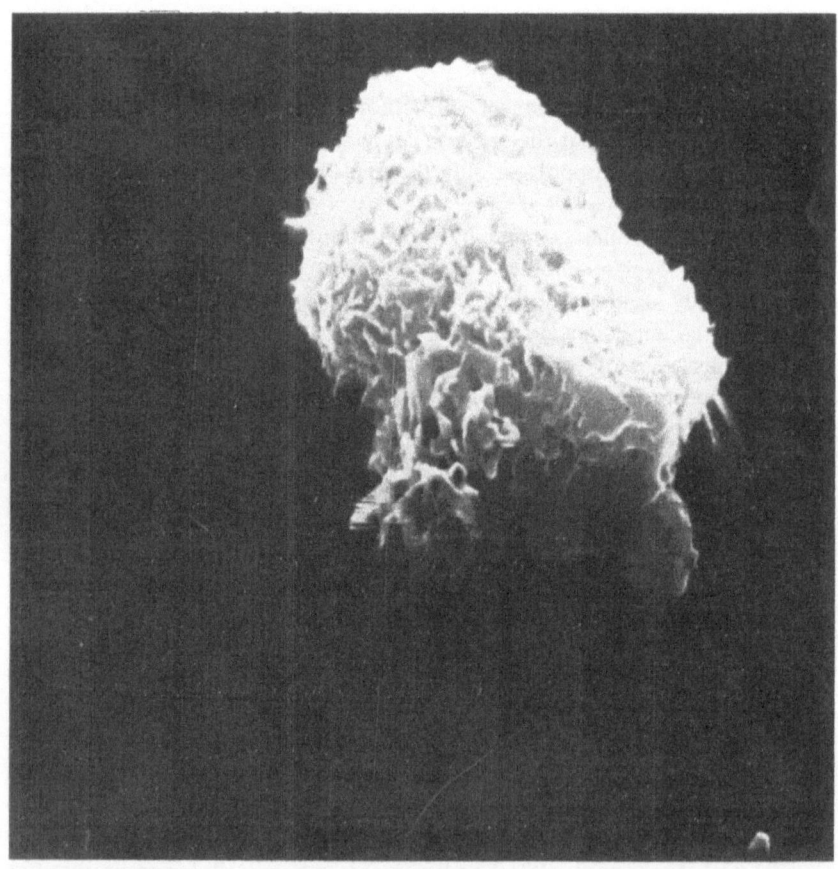

Fig. 75. Rounded cell shapes. Two keratocytes back to back. Scanning electron microscopy (x 3050).

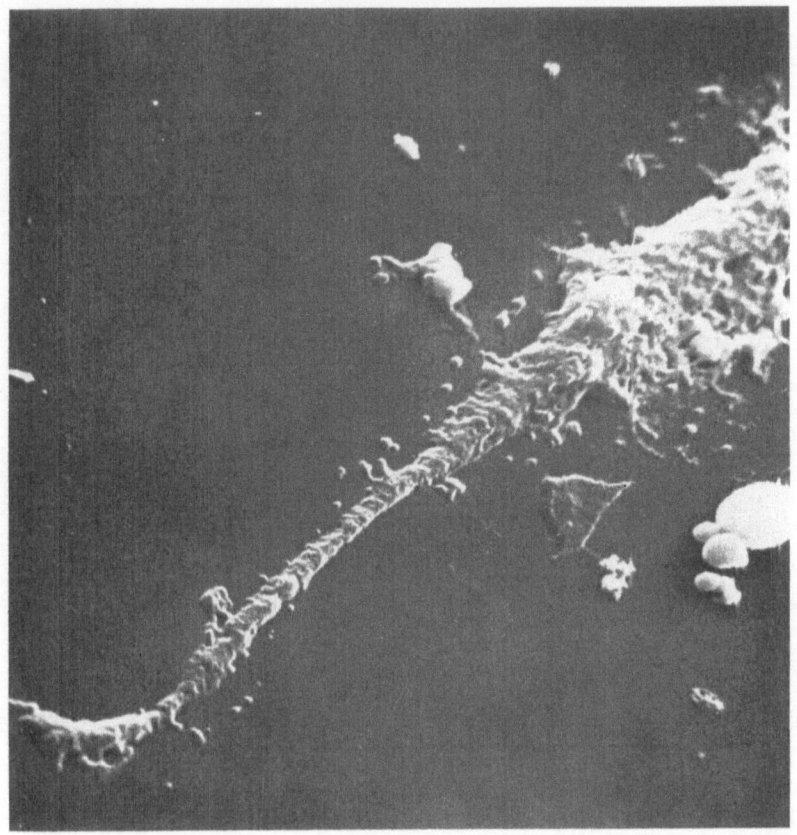

Fig. 76. Very long first-order pseudopodium. Its surface is anfractuous. Scanning electron microscopy (x 1225).

CONCLUSIONS

The scanning electron microscope shows:
1. Irregular cells and numerous cell debris, due to the rupture of pathological elements.
2. Numerous globular cells which are never seen in cultures of normal keratocytes.
3. The separation of certain parts of the cell body, giving rise to isolated elements.
4. An irregular cellular surface.

CHAPTER XIV

VITAL STAINING OF THE LYSOSOMES IN NORMAL KERATOCYTES AND IN KERATOCYTES FROM MACULAR DYSTROPHY

INTRODUCTION

It has been established that many basic or neutral substances can be fixed on the lysosomes of living cells (Koenig, 1963a and b; Allison et al., 1964a; Robbins et al., 1964; Allison et al., 1965a and b; Bastos et al., 1966; Zelenin, 1966; Barrett et al., 1968; Allison et al., 1973; Dingle et al., 1973b). Among these substances, there are fluorescent dyes, anti-inflammatory agents, cancerogenic products (Allison et al., 1964a) and some highly positively charged metals (Allison et al., 1966; Goldfischer, 1967; Allison et al., 1973) (Fig. 8).

Among the fluorescent dyes, the aminoacridines (euchrisine, acridine orange, quinacrine) must be mentioned. Some of these aminoacridines are fixed by the lysosomes and the cell nucleus (acridine orange and euchrisine), others only by the lysosomes (quinacrine) and others again only by the cell nucleus (acriflavine) (Allison et al., 1964c and 1973).

Acridine orange is the vital dye of choice. In the living cells of tissue cultures:

1. It stains the lysosomes selectively, giving them a red fluorescence (metachromatic staining);

2. It stains also the mitochondria, giving them a green fluorescence (orthochromatic staining);

3. Finally, it stains the nucleic acids of the nucleus, the DNA green and the RNA orange.

The vital staining depends essentially on the concentration of the dye and the optimal staining time.

When the cells have been fixed, acridine orange stains only the nucleic acids.

When the living cells have been stained with acridine orange and are then exposed to light of appropriate wavelength for an apropriate period of time, they undergo changes due to the 'photodynamic' effect.

We investigated the vital staining by acridine orange, of cultures of normal keratocytes and keratocytes from macular dystrophy.

PERSONAL OBSERVATIONS

We were the first to apply the techniques of vital lysosome staining in experimental ophthalmology.

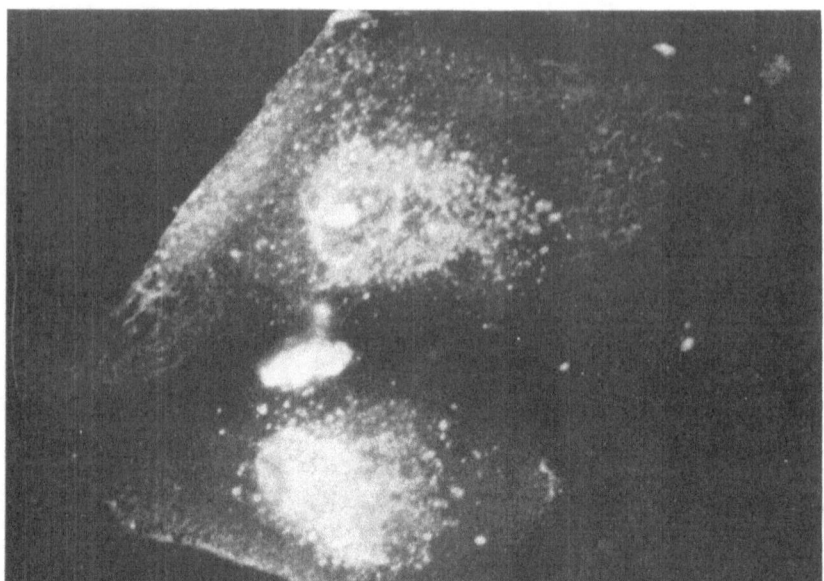

Fig. 77. Normal keratocytes. Two cells in a field of keratocytes. Lysosomes of various sizes are seen, grouped around the nucleus and also at the periphery. The nucleolus shows an orange fluorescence. Fluororescence microscopy (x 20 obj.).

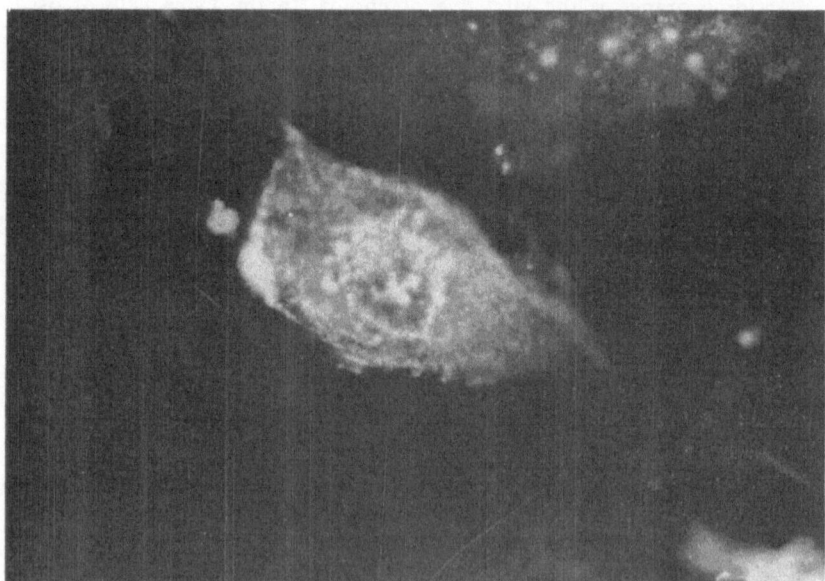

Fig. 78. Normal keratocytes. In these keratocytes, the lysosomes are arranged like a hat on the nucleus. The green fluorescent DNA of the caryoplasm is visible, as is also the orange fluorescence of the nucleolus. Fluorescence microscopy (x 20 obj.).

162

I. NORMAL KERATOCYTES

The following characteristics were seen in normal cultivated keratocytes, which had been incubated for eight minutes at 37°C in a solution of acridine orange at the concentration of $1:10^{-5}$ W/V, and which were then examined at the fluorescence microscope, using a dark-field condenser.

At low magnification the cytoplasm was seen to contain orangish granulations (Figs. 77 and 78), the staining being more red, and consequently more metachromatic, in the grouped cells than in the isolated ones.

At higher magnification, the *nucleus* showed a more or less homogeneous green fluorescence. The hue and the intensity of the fluorescence varied from one cell to another. In many cases the fluorescence was stronger at the periphery of the nucleus and at the level of the nuclear membrane (Fig. 79).

Each nucleus contained one to three nucleoli whose staining ranged from orange to yellow. The fluorescence of these nucleoli was not homogeneous. There were, indeed, areas more orange and more fluorescent than others. However, the whole nucleolus was fluorescent, which was demonstrated by comparing the fluorescent picture with that seen at the phase-contrast or the optical microscope after staining with toluidine blue.

The fluorescent staining of the nucleus corresponded exactly to that obtained in the fixed cells stained by acridine orange. In this case, as we have already stated, only the nucleic acids were stained: the RNA in orange-red, the DNA in green.

The cytoplasm, the background of which was not stained after eight minutes when a weak dye concentration was used, showed granules with an orange-red fluorescence and others with a green fluorescence.

1. The *granules with an orange-red fluorescence* corresponded to lysosomes (Figs. 77 to 80). They were particularly numerous and agglomerated near one pole and, in some cases, near the two poles of the nucleus. Their shape was mostly rounded, but in the fusiform cells, they could display a more elongated shape, following the longest cell axis, because of the compression of the lysosomes by the tonofibrils. In general, they were brighter as the nucleus was approached.

Their dimensions were very variable:

a. There were punctiform lysosomes measuring less than 0.5 μm and filling the ectoplasm;

b. Medium-sized lysosomes measuring from 0.5 to 1.5 μm, less numerous and in many cases grouped near one pole of the nucleus;

c. Large lysosomes measuring from 1.5 to 3 μm, not exceeding four to eight in number.

There was no relationship between the size of the granule and its fluorescent spectrum, which ranged from red to orange. On the other hand, the

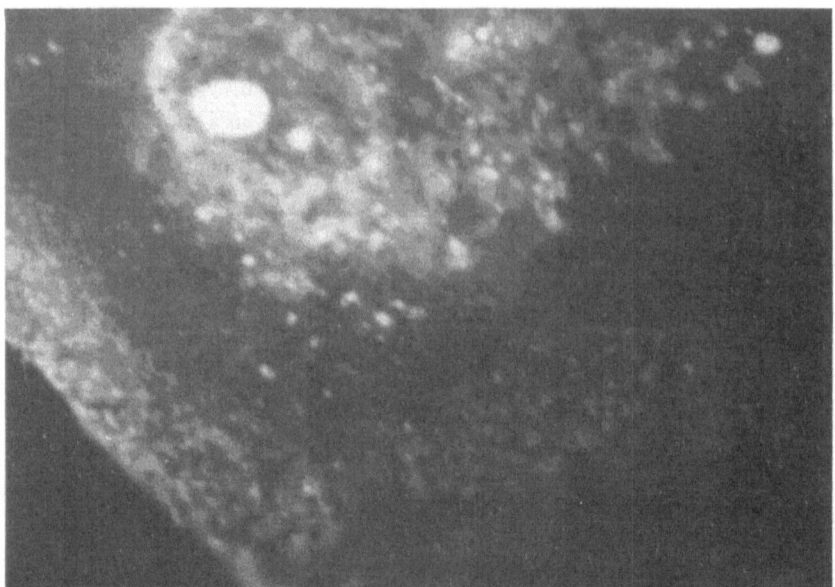

Fig. 79. Normal keratocyte. Orange-fluorescent lysosomes mixed with very numerous mitochondria having a dark-green fluorescence are visible around the nucleus. The RNA of the nucleolus is highly fluorescent. Fluorescence microscopy (x 100 obj.).

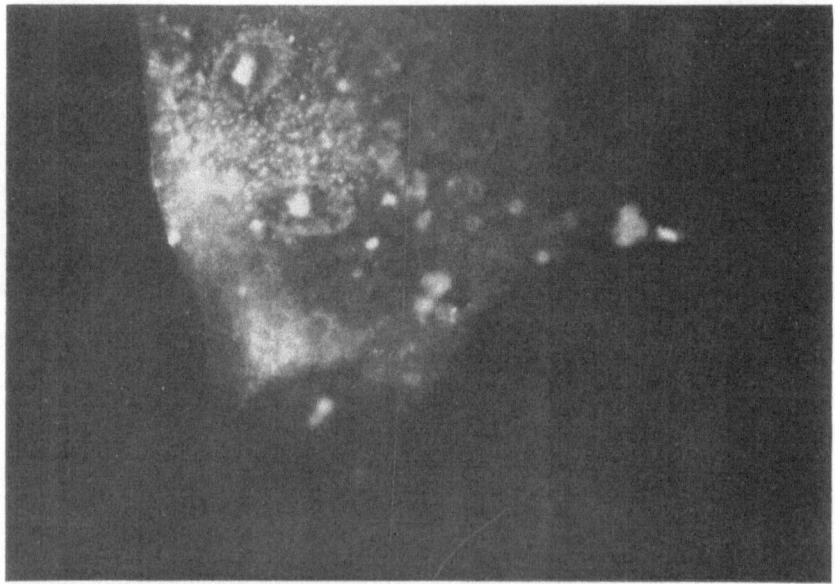

Fig. 80. Normal keratocytes. Immediately after the cell division, the lysosomes group themselves between the two nuclei, in a cytoplasm common to the two cells. Fluorescence microscopy (x 20 obj.).

intensity of the fluorescence diminished from the largest lysosomes to the smallest ones.

Lysosomes of medium sizes were frequently found in the pseudopodia of the cells.

In some cells, granulated areas measuring 10 to 12 μm were found, located against the cytoplasmic membrane. The individuality of these granules was less well defined, possibly because they were less well agglomerated. In some cases the cellular membrane displayed a yellow fluorescence.

Comparative microscopical studies showed that all the granules appearing black at the phase-contrast microscope and bright at the dark-field microscope, took the acridine orange and were positively stained by the Takeuchi and Tanoue method for acid phosphatase. In other words, they were lysosomes.

The punctiform granules were not visible at the phase-contrast microscope. However, they were positively stained by the Takeuchi and Tanoue method and therefore, they also were lysosomes.

The peripheral fluorescent clots were not stained by this method, but were positive for reticulin.

2. *Granules with a green fluorescence* were always found. These elongated elements measured from 0.5 to 1 μm and numbered between five and ten. The intensity of the green fluorescence was lower than that of the lysosomes. These granules were mitochondria, as they were also stained by Janus green, which is a specific dye for mitochondria.

Cell division

During the cell division, a reorganisation and a redistribution of the lysosomes were observed. This phenomenon was more obvious if vitamin-A at a concentration of 1000 to 3000 IU per millilitre of culture medium, was added to the culture medium, and if afterwards the vital staining with acridine orange was effected by mounting the monolayer with the same solution containing the fluorochrome.

Repeated, but very short observations (in order to prevent the photodynamic effect) showed small lysosomes spreaded at the periphery of the cells. Thereafter the lysosomes could no longer be found, although a greenish background fluorescence could still be observed. When the nucleus divided, the lysosomes reappeared, occupying the cytoplasm, which was still common to the two new nuclei (Fig. 80). They were small or medium-sized lysosomes, located in the internuclear area. Finally, the lysosomes migrated, half to each cell, and reached the juxtanuclear area of the daughter cells. There were sometimes three nuclei with an apparently common cytoplasm, where the lysosomes were arranged in a triangular area, of which the apices corresponded to the three nuclei. It was only at the end of the cell division that lysosomes of larger sizes were seen to appear.

If acid phosphatase was stained before and during this process, it was seen that, right at the beginning of the cell division, the unfixed cells showed a positive staining, indicating an increase in the permeability of the lysosomal membrane. Vitamin-A stimulates this process, because it renders the membrane more fragile and so facilitates the cell division.

On the other hand, if prednisone, in a concentration of 1000 to 3000 IU per millilitre of culture medium, was added to the culture medium, the number of lysosomes did not change, and did not fuse anymore. The prednisone strengthens the lysosomal membrane and consequently stops the growth of the culture by inhibiting the cell division.

Dynamics of the vital staining

Staining for one to two minutes with acridine orange at 10 μg/ml (1:10^5 W/V) showed a marked green fluorescence of the cytoplasm. Some granules were seen, which took on a more intense green or a yellow fluorescence. The fluorescence of the nucleus was green or, on the contrary, absent. The orange fluorescence that appeared first was, in general, that of the nucleoli. Vacuoles of pinocytosis were also seen (Fig. 81); they measured from 2 to 3 μm. The dye contained in these vacuoles was of a more intense green than that of the cytoplasmic fluorescence.

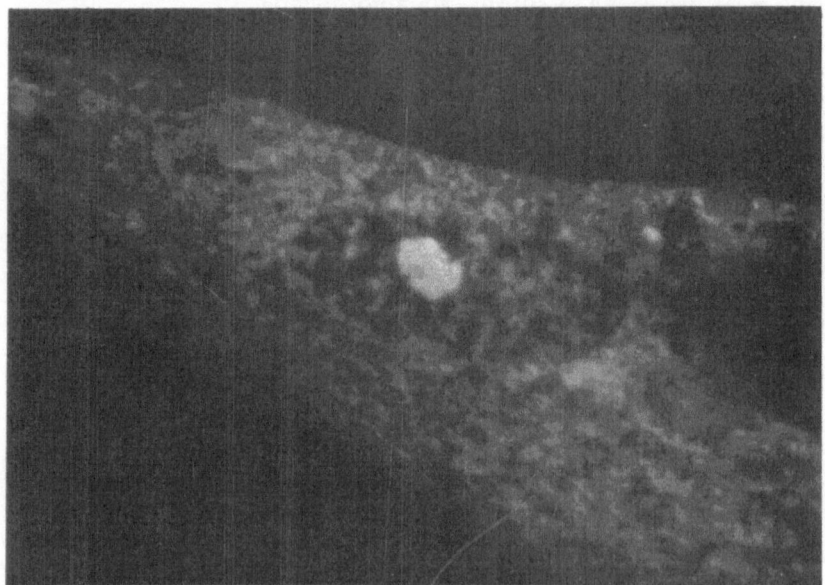

Fig. 81. Normal keratocyte. At the beginning of the vital staining, numerous vacuoles of pinocytosis can be observed at the periphery of the cell. They show a dark-green fluorescence. Fluorescence microscopy (x 50 obj.).

166

Staining for two to five minutes showed a red fluorescence, which appeared in the granules and was the highest in the nucleoli. The green fluorescence of the cytoplasm disappeared. The number of stained lysosomes increased. Vacuoles of pinocytosis with green fluorescence were still seen.

Staining for five to eight minutes gave the maximum result, both for the orange-red fluorescence of the lysosomes and for the green fluorescence of the mitochondria.

Staining for fifteen to twenty minutes did not change the results.

If acridine orange at a stronger concentration was used (50 μg/ml), the fluorescence of the lysosomes, the nucleoli and the cytoplasm was stronger.

If the dye was used at 100 μg/ml, a homogeneous red fluorescence of the cytoplasm, an orange staining of the nucleus and an intense red staining of the nucleoli were observed after one minute.

When the cells were washed two or three times in a medium that did not contain acridine orange, and if they were then incubated at 37°C for twenty minutes in a normal culture medium, the orange-red fluorescence of the lysosomes was seen to appear again, because of the disappearance of the excess staining of the background.

The green fluorescence of the cytoplasmic background could be obtained after three minutes of staining at 37°C with 10 μg/ml acridine orange. The green fluorescence of the DNA and the red fluorescence of the RNA were obtained under the same conditions. Even a longer staining did not show the fluorescence of the lysosomes. If the concentration of the dye was increased, the background fluorescence became more red, but did not concentrate in the lysosomes.

If weaker concentrations of acridine-orange were used (less than 5 μg/ml), it was necessary to increase the incubation time, in order to obtain the desired result.

II. KERATOCYTES IN MACULAR DYSTROPHY

The keratocytes in macular dystrophy were very polymorphic. In order to obtain a good result, it was necessary to use acridine orange at 20-100 μg/ml and to increase the incubation time up to fifteen minutes.

Many of the cells showed a pale and homogeneous greenish fluorescence (Fig. 82). They were considered to be non-viable.

The viable cells contained a *nucleus*, which was in some cases normal and in others deteriorated. In the caryoplasm, clumps with greenish-yellow fluorescence were seen. These clumps were often located against the nuclear membrane, which then displayed the same fluorescence. This situation was similar to that of prepicnosis.

The nucleoli were mostly normal, although their fluorescence might in some cases be more yellowish.

It might happen that the nucleus became smaller, showing a uniform red or yellow fluorescence.

The *cytoplasm* contained lysosomes of variable appearance (Figs. 82, 83 and 84). The rounded cells contained large lysosomes measuring from 2 to 5 μm, whose red or orange fluorescence was very bright. The racket-shaped cells contained lysosomes measuring from 2 to 4 μm, occupying all the cytoplasm, or only the area neighbouring a nuclear pole. The fusiform cells displayed lysosomes of three types: rod-like lysosomes from 2 to 4 μm in length and from 1 to 2 μm in width, rounded, apparently normal lysosomes, which were nevertheless too large, and finally single giant lysosomes occupying a whole pole of the cell. All these lysosomes showed a very bright orange-red fluorescence.

It might happen that all the cytoplasm became uniformly red. This phenomenon was probably due to an excessive staining of normal lysosomes, the concentration of the dye being too high and the incubation time too long.

In some cases, the distribution of the lysosomes was reversed. They were found at the periphery of the cytoplasm, whereas the centre was occupied by mitochondria.

All these lysosomes were positive for acid phosphatase. Nevertheless, those whose size exceeded 3 or 4 μm, took on the appearance of vacuoles at

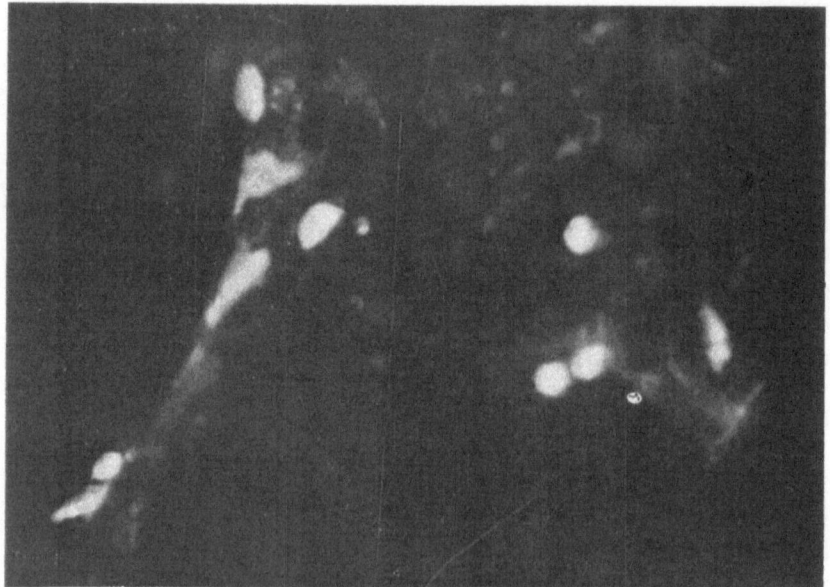

Fig. 82. Macular dystrophy of the cornea. Numerous dead cells with a dark-green fluorescence form a meshwork. Very irregular small cells with orange cytoplasm are arranged on this meshwork. Fluorescence microscopy (x 100 obj.).

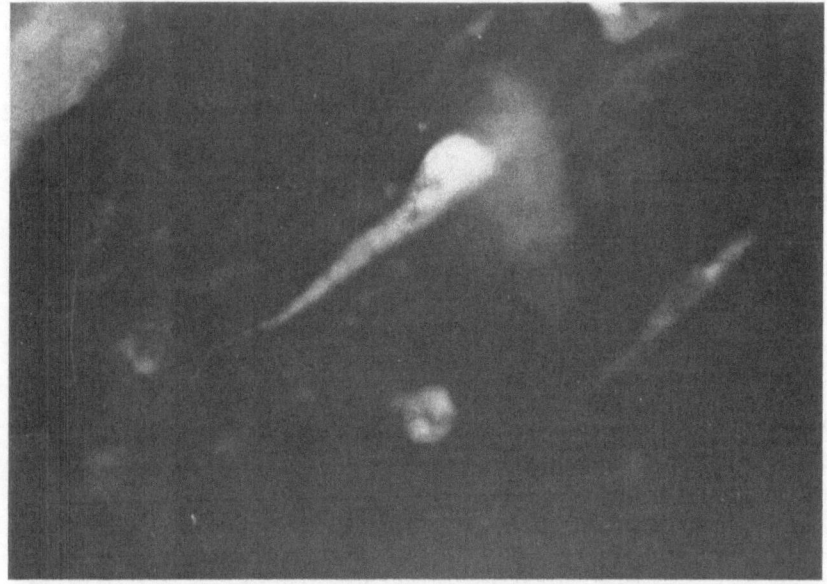

Fig. 83. Macular dystrophy of the cornea. Small fusiform cell, one pole of which is occupied by orange fluorescence. Fluorescence microscopy (× 20 obj.).

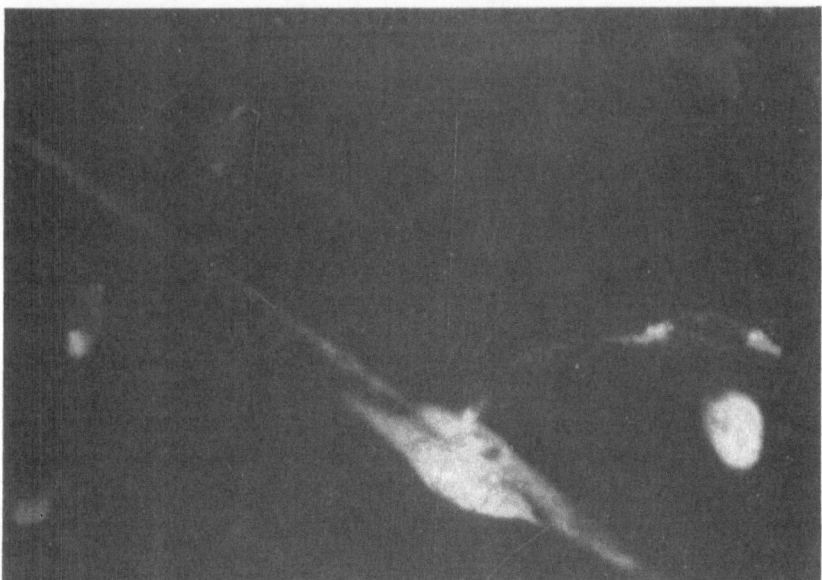

Fig. 84. Macular dystrophy of the cornea. Two fusiform cells, one of them being binuclear and rounded. The shape of the lysosomes is ill-defined, but a homogeneous orange fluorescence is visible in some places. Fluorescence microscopy (× 20 obj.).

169

the phase-contrast microscope. Some granules and vacuoles were stained metachromatically by toluidine blue, and positively by other dyes for mucopolysaccharides.

In many cases, groups of rounded degenerating cells with a bright, orange fluorescence, were observed.

The mitochondria had a normal appearance, but their number and their distribution were very variable.

The *cell division* took place in cells having a more normal appearance. The lysosomes then behaved as in normal keratocytes.

Dynamics of the vital staining in keratocytes
from macular dystrophy

When acridine orange was used at a concentration of 10 μg/ml (1:10^5 W/V), the cells showed only a weak uniform green fluorescence. Even after fifteen minutes of incubation, the fluorescence was still ill defined.

At a higher concentration (50-100 μg/ml), the optimum staining time was fifteen to twenty minutes. The staining was then progressive. There was first a uniform greenish fluorescence which afterwards concentrated in the lysosomes. They displayed at first a yellowish fluorescence, which later changed to red. The nuclei were stained more slowly, as were the nucleoli, which showed at first a yellow fluorescence.

CONCLUSIONS

The mechanism of the vital staining by acridine orange is explained in Figure 8.

The lysosomes of the keratocytes in tissue culture are revealed by the vital staining with acridine orange, which gives them an orange-red fluorescence.

In *normal keratocytes*, the lysosomes, which are characterised by a positivity of the staining for acid phosphatase, are mostly grouped around one or both of the poles of the nucleus. It is possible to distinguish three types of lysosomes, according to the size of the granules, which may, indeed, measure less than 0.5 μm, between 0.5 and 1.5 μm or more than 1.5 μm. The acridine orange positive granules correspond to most of the black granules observed at the phase-contrast microscope, but not to all of them. There are, moreover, at the cell periphery some fluorescent clots positively stained by the Wilder method. These reticulin clots are the precursors of collagen. Finally, the acridine orange gives a green fluorescence to the mitochondria, which can also be stained specifically by Janus green.

At the onset of cell division, there is a sensibilisation of the lysosomal membrane, with diffusion of the fluorochrome toward the cytoplasm. After

170

the nuclear division, there is a redistribution of the lysosomes in the daughter-cells, the lysosomes occupying first the internuclear area. Finally, they are grouped around one nuclear pole.

The blue part of the spectrum has a 'photodynamic' effect, which vacuolises the cytoplasm, deteriorates the nucleus and detaches the cells from the monolayer surface.

In *keratocytes of macular dystrophy*, numerous changes are observed. A higher dye concentration and a longer incubation time are necessary to stain the lysosomes, which take the most various shapes, ranging from the normal up to the giant shape, which occupies an entire pole of the cell. Most of the lysosomes are large, measuring from 2 to 4 μm. In short, there is a hypertrophy of the lysosomal system, which tends to compensate the enzymatic deficiency without being capable of achieving it.

CHAPTER XV

ACTIVE BIOLOGICAL SUBSTANCE PRESENT IN NORMAL KERATOCYTES AND CAPABLE OF ACTING ON THE STORED MUCOPOLYSACCHARIDES IN MACULAR DYSTROPHY OF THE CORNEA

PERSONAL OBSERVATIONS

We found an active biological substance (an enzyme or an enzymatic complex), which is capable of acting on the acid mucopolysaccharides (keratosulphate) stored in macular dystrophy of the cornea.

I. EXPERIMENT

1. Keratocyte cultures were hypotonised by means of 0.075 M potassium chloride for twenty to thirty minutes.
2. A pig's corneal stroma was homogenised and 0.075 M potassium chloride was added, the solvent being allowed to act for thirty minutes.
3. Sections obtained from two different cases of macular dystrophy of the cornea were incubated for three hours at 38°C with either the homogenate of normal keratocyte culture or the homogenate of normal corneal stroma, the active substance being probably soluble.
4. By way of control, we incubated sections with only the solvent which had been used in the preparation of the homogenate.

The sections were divided into three groups: the first group of three sections treated with the homogenate of normal corneal stroma, the second group of three sections treated with the homogenate of a normal keratocyte culture and the third group of three sections treated with the solvent alone. Each section was stained by dyes for mucopolysaccharides.

II. RESULTS

Staining with toluidine blue showed that the sections treated with the homogenate of a normal keratocyte culture or of normal corneal stroma were stained orthochromatically, whereas those treated with the solvent alone were stained metachromatically.

The staining with colloidal iron and Alcian blue was negative in the sections treated with corneal homogenates, whereas it remained positive in the sections treated with the solvent alone (Figs. 85 and 86).

We observed also that, by adding a piece of normal cornea to a culture of keratocytes obtained from macular dystrophy, the growth of the pathological keratocytes was accelerated.

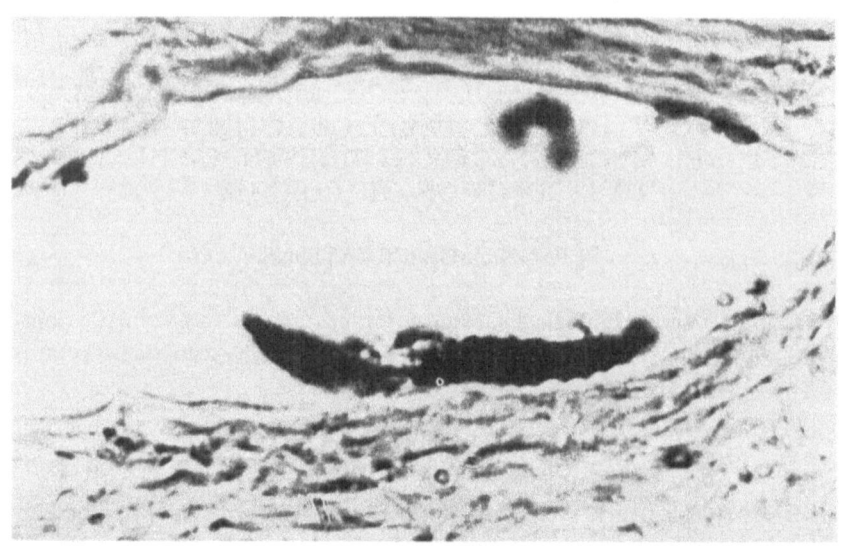

Fig. 85. Staining of Rinehart and Abul-Haj. Keratocyte whose cytoplasm is completely filled with mucopolysaccharides, the nucleus being scarcely visible (× 1000 obj.).

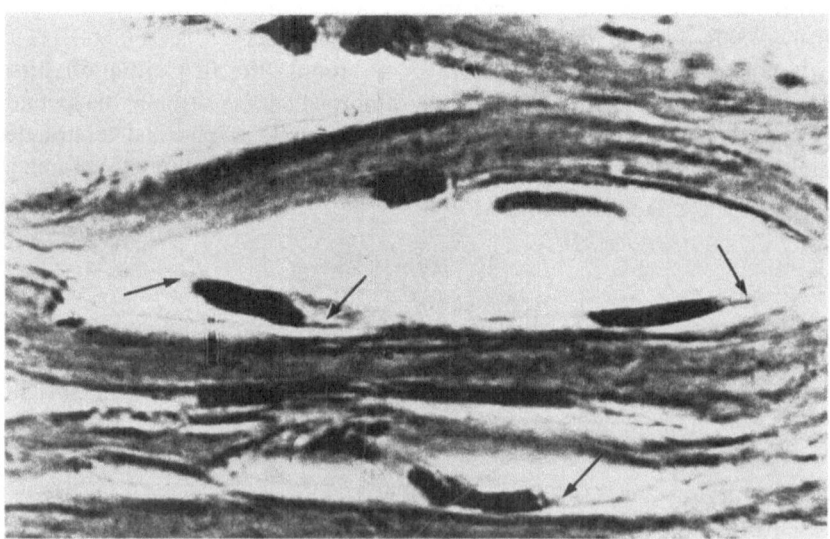

Fig. 86. Staining of Rinehart and Abul-Haj. The section was treated with an extract of normal keratocytes, obtained from three culture flasks of the same strain. The arrows indicate the cytoplasm which no longer contains mucopolysaccharides (× 1000 obj.).

A histochemical study of the lysosomal enzymes, in accordance with the techniques described in Chapter I, indicated that there existed a deficiency of β-glucuronidase in the pathological cells.

We made the counter-proof by examining the action of β-glucuronidase on frozen histological sections. The enzyme negatived the stainings for acid mucopolysaccharides as well as the metachromasia due to toluidine blue at pH 6.

DISCUSSION AND CONCLUSIONS

Our experiments show that there exists, in fresh corneal tissue and more particularly in fresh keratocytes, an active substance which is capable of neutralising the mucopolysaccharides stored in macular dystrophy of the cornea. The substance is obtained by preparing homogenates with a hypotonising solvent, which does not contain this active substance. Consequently the latter must therefore be of cellular origin.

Jones et al. (1961) showed that the mucopolysaccharides of macular dystrophy are not sensitive to hyaluronidase. This enzyme exists in the primary cell lysosomes, with other mucopolysaccharidic enzymes, namely α-glucosidase, β-N-acetylglucosaminidase, β-glucuronidase, β-galactosidase, α-monosidase, β-xilosidase, arylsulphatase and neurominidase (Wattiaux, 1969).

In our experiments, the active substance may very well be an enzyme contained in the lysosomes, since it is obtained by adding a hypotonising solvent that breaks down the lysosomal membranes.

We could demonstrate the absence, in the pathological cultures, of β-glucuronidase, which is present in the normal control cultures. On the other hand, β-glucuronidase negatives the mucopolysaccharidic deposits of the macular dystrophy of the cornea in the histological sections.

175

CHAPTER XVI

PATHOGENESIS OF MACULAR DYSTROPHY
OF THE CORNEA

Macular dystrophy of the cornea is an hereditary disorder which is transmitted as an autosomal recessive trait. It is characterised by the storage of acid mucopolysaccharides in the corneal stroma (keratosulphate). Unlike the generalised mucopolysaccharidoses with corneal involvement (Goldberg et al., 1965), macular dystrophy is a localised disorder, probably because the type of enzyme involved is exclusive to the cornea.

At the present time it is known that the mucopolysaccharides are synthesised by the Golgi's apparatus of the mesodermal cells, which, depending upon their degree of differentiation and their genetic messages, produce a particular mucopolysaccharidic 'pool'. It is so that the keratocytes produce above all keratosulphate, the hyalocytes above all hyaluronic acid and so on (Peterson et al., 1964; Neutra et al., 1966; Rambourg et al., 1969; Revel, 1970).

The mucopolysaccharides are catabolised by enzymes contained in the lysosomes (Dingle, 1972; Dingel et al., 1973b), which were discovered by De Duve and his co-workers in 1949 (De Duve, 1973).

The fundamental characteristic of the lysosomes is the membrane in which they are enclosed. Their enzyme content has a much more acid pH (less than 5) than the other components of the cell.

The lysosomes constitute a cell compartment which contains enzymes capable of catabolising: (1) proteins, (2) certain lipids and (3) carbohydrates.

The lysosomes are individualised, from both the histochemical and the cytochemical points of view, by the presence of acid phosphatase, which is now considered as the lysosome marker.

The mucopolysaccharides would be catabolised in the secondary lysosomes, thanks to the enzymes contained in the primary lysosomes and synthesised in the endoplasmic reticulum (Fig. 87), the energy for the process being supplied by the mitochondrion.

The accumulation of mucopolysaccharides in a cell may be due to the following:

1. An *excess of production*. Our studies on tissue cultures, as well as the hypertrophy of the Golgi's apparatus observed *in vivo* and *in vitro*, show that this factor plays a role. The hyperproduction is also due to a hyper-

plasia of the keratocytes. In normal cells, however, the hyperproduction of mucopolysaccharides is compensated by the hyperfunction of a complete catabolic system. In the keratocytes of macular dystrophy of the cornea, whether *in vivo* or *in vitro*, the lysosomal system is hypertrophied, but its catabolic system is incomplete, since it lacks one or, perhaps, more enzymes.

2. A *catabolic deficiency*. This fact was demonstrated by Cotlier et al. (1972), who found a deficiency of α-galactosidase in the lysosomes. For our part, we demonstrated the absence of β-glucuronidase in the cases we examined. It is, consequently, possible that two different enzyme deficiencies can produce macular dystrophy of the cornea. It must, nevertheless, be noted

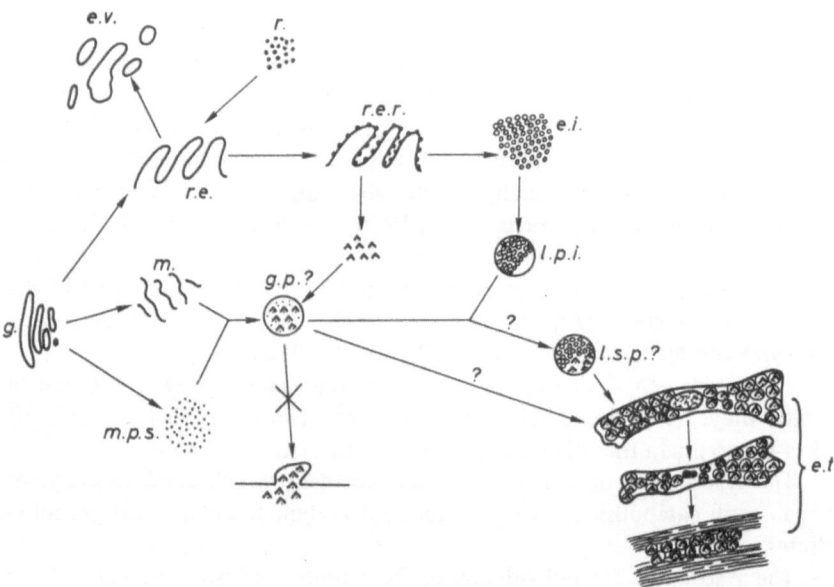

Fig. 87. Pathogenic diagram of macular dystrophy of the cornea. The Golgi's apparatus (g.) synthesises the mucopolysaccharides (m.p.s.) and forms the membranes (m.). From these two elements the granules of mucopolysaccharides (g.p.) are formed. In addition, the Golgi's apparatus produces the endoplasmic reticulum (r.e.) and the vacuolar spaces (e.v.). The endoplasmic reticulum forms, with the ribosomes, the ribosomal endoplasmic reticulum (r.e.r.), which synthesises the lysosomal enzymes (e.i.), some of which are missing, so that the primary lysosomes (l.p.i.) will be incomplete. On the other hand, the ribosomal endoplasmic reticulum (r.e.r.) can give rise to a protein, which will contribute to the formation of the mucopolysaccharidic granule (g.p.). By the fusion of the incomplete primary lysosome (l.p.i.) and the mucopolysaccharidic granule (g.p.) are formed the secondary lysosomes (l.s.p.), in which the digestion of the acid mucopolysaccharides cannot occur. The storage of these occurs then in three stages (accumulation of the mucopolysaccharides with pycnosis and cellular death, followed by interlamellar deposit).

178

that the methods used by Cotlier and by us are different, one being chemical and the other histochemical.

3. It is probable that the deterioration of the mitochondria also plays a role in the disturbance of the dynamic equilibrium of the mucopolysaccharides. These mitochondria must, indeed, supply the energy necessary for the metabolic processes.

4. The phagocytosis of free mucopolysaccharides in the stroma can also play a role (Jones et al., 1959). We were able to demonstrate that normal keratocytes possess *in vitro* a great capacity of phagocytosis (François et al., 1973). However, that phenomenon is not a primary one, as in the cultures of pathological keratocytes, the newformed cells, which are far from the specimen, containing the mucopolysaccharides to be phagocyted, show also a storage.

The storage develops progressively in the keratocytes (Klintworth et al., 1964; Seitz et al., 1965; Jones et al., 1961; Payrau et al., 1967; Teng, 1966; Morgan, 1966; Lorenzetti et al., 1967; Garner, 1969; Hermann et al., 1971; Thiel et al., 1971; François et al., 1972c; Blümcke et al., 1972; Malbran, 1972; Malbran et al., 1973; François et al., 1975a and b). The material shows the histochemical reactions characteristic of keratosulphate. Garner (1969) analysed the interlamellar substance obtained from destroyed keratocytes and found that it is a mucoid rich in hexose and desoxyhexose, in keratosulphate without hyaluronic acid, in chondroitin-4-sulphate and chondroitin-6-sulphate,

François et al. (1975b) showed the possibility of an accumulation of mucopolysaccharides due to a hereditary metabolic disturbance, but secondarily linked to the production of mucopolysaccharides.

We can describe four histological stages in the development of the storage by the keratocytes (Figs. 42, 43, 44 and 45):

Stage I. Some mucopolysaccharide granules are observed in the cytoplasm, the nucleus being normal. At the electron microscope, the cellular membrane is seen to be intact.

Stage II. The mucopolysaccharides accumulate, and the cell becomes globular. The nucleus remains more or less normal. At the electron microscope, a complete cytoplasmic membrane is seen, although reformed in some places, after the escape of some granulations.

Stage III. The cell retains its shape, but the nucleus is picnotic. At the electron microscope, numerous ruptures of the cellular membrane are visible.

Stage IV. The nucleus has disappeared and only an interlamellar deposit remains.

During all these stages, the acid phosphatase reaction is positive in the granules.

In the keratocytes, there is also an anarchic fusion among the membranes

179

of the various structures. The fusion between the lysosomes and the endoplasmic reticulum may be observed, what gives rise to dilated cisterns containing a wide variety of materials.

The extracellular deposits (Jones et al., 1961) which are found in the stroma, are of two types:

a. Interlamellar deposits (Teng, 1966; François et al., 1972c), which originate from the keratocytes, their cytoplasmic and lysosomal origin being demonstrated by the presence of acid phosphatases. In addition, the electron microscope shows that these deposits contain the same elements as these found within the cells. They correspond to Stage IV of the cell storage.

b. The lesions of the lamellae show progressive stages of destruction, due to the catabolic enzymes of the lysosomes originating from the ruptured keratocytes. It is proved by the positivity of the acid phosphatase test. We know, moreover, that the lysosomes contain the enzymatic 'pool' capable of catabolising the stromal constituents.

Studies at the polarisation microscope show also the progressive destruction of the stroma (François et al., 1972c; pers. obs.). The lamellar deposits consist of deteriorated, basophil and transversely oriented collagen. They constitute a dense crystalline structure (François et al., 1972c), which could be due to a delay in the reabsorption of the stroma by the cells.

On the other hand, Teng (1966) thinks that the lysosomes would be activated by the intracytoplasmic accumulation of mucopolysaccharides. The rupture of the lysosomes would liberate acid hydrolases, which would cause the destruction of the cell and their diffusion in the neighbouring stroma. This hypothesis is confirmed by the optical polarisation studies of François et al. (1972c).

We found the following changes of the lysosomes:

1. *In vitro, primary changes* are observed, developing immediately after cellular division.

2. The shape and the arrangement of the lysosomes are abnormal. Moreover, there are giant lysosomes.

3. At the electron microscope, the lysosomes show in many cases incomplete membranes. Fusions between the lysosomal membrane and those of other structures can also be found.

4. The lysosomes are functionally deficient, because, in spite of their number, they are unable to catabolise the mucopolysaccharides produced by the cell.

According to Teng (1966), the mucopolysaccharides accumulate first in the endoplasmic reticulum. We think, however, that they accumulate from the onset of the disease, and that it is only after the fusion between the mucopolysaccharidic granules and the membranes of the endoplasmic reticulum that they are found in the latter. The mucopolysaccharides must be in impermeable compartments, independent of the endoplasmic reticulum, as this reticulum synthesises the collagen, which precipitates *in situ*, when it is in presence of mucopolysaccharides.

That is precisely what happens *in vitro*, where large spaces in the endoplasmic reticulum contain collagen precipitated in the form of long spacing fibres.

The intra- and extra-cellular deposits, consisting of a material with a periodicity of 120 Å, are probably due to hydrolysis of the stroma by lysosomal enzymes and to their reprecipitation by liberated mucopolysaccharides.

In Chapter X we have seen that the changes of the epithelium and the endothelium are secondary (Figs. 55, 59, 60, 61a and b, 62 and 63). Snip et al. (1973), however, think that macular dystrophy is a primary disorder of the endothelium.

The opacities observed clinically consist of mucopolysaccharidic deposits, which, thanks to their hydrophilia, attract water and are surrounded by a halo of oedema.

Figure 87 shows the pathogenesis of macular dystrophy of the cornea.

CHAPTER XVII

TREATMENT OF MACULAR DYSTROPHY OF THE CORNEA

a. There is no *medical treatment* for macular dystrophy of the cornea. It is possible that an enzymatic therapy, applied early, might be effective because the mucopolysaccharidic deposits are sensitive to the catabolic enzymes present in normal keratocytes. However, it might be that these enzymes, acting for a long time, would deteriorate the normal mucopolysaccharidic structures of the stroma.

b. *Surgical treatment.* Although lamellar keratoplasty could bring about some improvement, the fact that the posterior limiting membrane is also affected, makes it necessary to perform a perforating keratoplasty, the more so that at the electron microscope or at the scanning microscope lesions are seen in cases wherein the posterior limiting membrane seems clinically normal. Malbran (1972) and Malbran et al. (1973) recommend a keratoplasty of 7.5 to 8 mm, which gives excellent results. As the endothelium is frequently, although subclinically invaded, a corneal graft with a good endothelial viability (at least 80%) should be used.

Recurrences are nevertheless possible (Keates et al., 1965; Klintworth et al., 1964; Morgan, 1966; Lorenzetti et al., 1967). This possibility is also a contra-indication for lamellar keratoplasty, because it is impossible to remove all the affected stroma (Malbran, 1972; Malbran et al., 1973).

Since the disorder is a primary storage of the keratocytes, it is probable that the recurrences are due to a proliferation of the genetically pathological keratocytes of the host cornea, which invade the graft.

The recurrences, however, occur only tardily (five years in a case of Malbran and Victoria-Troncoso, 1973). The opacities appear at the level of the ring separating the graft and the host cornea, and thereafter extend toward the centre (Malbran, 1972; Malbran et al., 1973). In the case of a lamellar keratoplasty, the greater the area of contact between the graft and the host, the more probable an early recurrence (Malbran, 1972; Malbran et al., 1973).

SUMMARY

Architectonically, the cornea is a lamellar structure, each lamella consisting of fascicles arranged at various angles.

In situ, the keratocytes are almost inactive cells. Nevertheless, they can be activated by a wound of the cornea and by tissue culture. That fact shows that they are highly differentiated cells, which are different from other cells of the connective tissue series.

As regards the activation of the keratocytes by corneal wound, we have observed the following:

During the first twenty-four hours, polynuclears, few in number and probably originating from the precorneal lacrimal film, invade the wound, during which slipping of the epithelial cells and their proliferation at the level of the incision are observed. As soon as the epithelisation is complete, the polynuclears disappear, and a connective proliferation is seen, setting in after forty-eight hours and pressing back the epithelial growth.

Already during the first twenty-four hours, the keratocytes distant 200 to 250 μm from the wound, which does not yet enclose keratocytes, show an active nucleus as a result of the increase in the number of the nucleoli, which varies from two to five. Furthermore, the volume of their cytoplasm increases. They take on, indeed, a star-shaped appearance, because of the shortening of their extensions. Finally, an increase in the number of keratosulphate granules is seen. This is the period of latency, during which there is yet no cellular proliferation.

After twenty-four to seventy-two hours, mitoses, which reach their maximum between the third and the fifth day, are observed. Most of the cells found at that moment in the wound, originate from the division of keratocytes, because 90% of these cells are characterised by the presence of keratosulphate granules.

These cells remain morphologically unchanged between the fifth and the fifteenth day. From that time onward, their number diminishes. Between the first and the third month, their cytoplasm and their nuclei regress.

At the electron microscope one can see, already after twenty-four hours, a progressive development of the organelles: Golgi's apparatus, mitochondria and dense corpuscles surrounded by a membrane, which are probably lysosomes. The cellular surface is rough, and from the third day, numerous electron-dense deposits adhere to the cellular membrane.

At the end of fifteen days, some cell atrophy is seen, although after three months active elements are still found.

The histochemical characteristics of the keratocytes activated by traumatism are identical with these of the keratocytes in tissue culture.

The principal fact is the increase of the number of intracytoplasmic mucopolysaccharidic granules observed already after twelve hours.

During the course of cicatrisation, several phases can be distinguished:
1. At the beginning there is an epithelial phase, wherein the lysosomal enzymes of the epithelium, including catabolic enzymes such as collagenase and those acting on the mucopolysaccharides, are liberated into the wound.
2. A phase of development of the enzymatic system of the keratocytes. This phase occupies the latency period. There is at that time an intense cellular biosynthesis, which becomes apparent after forty-eight hours, although the epithelial phase is still not finished.
3. A phase of biosynthesis of the mucopolysaccharides, which begins at the twenty-fourth hour.
4. A phase of cellular division, which starts after the forty-eigth hour.
5. A phase of fibrillogenesis, the extracellular product of which can be detected histochemically from the fifth day on.
6. A phase of organization, which continues until after the third month.
7. A phase of involution, which becomes apparent from the fifteenth day on.

All these phases overlap to a greater or lesser extent and can display variations.

As regards the keratocytes in tissue culture, the following may be observed:

Morphologically, a very active nucleus with two to five nucleoli is found, as well as cytoplasm containing vacuoles and peripheral and central granules.

Histochemically, it can be demonstrated that the granules contain keratosulphate. The peripheral granules contain in addition reticulin, which is stored in granules that are probably different from those enclosing the mucopolysaccharides. The vacuoles contain lipids.

Macular dystrophy of the cornea is a mucopolysaccharidosis localised to the cornea. The mucopolysaccharides, produced by the Golgi's apparatus, are stored in the cytoplasmic granules of the keratocytes. When the cell bursts, these granules invade the stroma. Histochemical methods, such as this of Saunders (1964), and the metachromatic curves prove that the stored product contains keratosulphate.

The keratocytes and the stromal lesions were studied at the transmission and scanning electron microscopes. Numerous particles of the lysosomal

186

type were found. The lesions are, indeed, positive for acid phosphatase, which is a lysosomal marker.

The cultures of corneas affected by macular dystrophy show:

a. That the storage is the result of a primary disorder of the keratocytes.
b. That the epithelial and endothelial lesions are secondary.
c. That the cells have a very short life-span.
d. That there is a very high lysosomal activity.

The tissue cultures made it also possible to study the behaviour of the cells *in vitro*. They were studied by various microscopical and histochemical methods.

The *in vitro* study of the lysosomes of the keratocytes by means of vital stainings with acridine orange at the fluorescence microscope shows their numerous alterations.

A substance present in the homogenates of cultures and of normal active corneas is capable of neutralising the stainings for mucopolysaccharides in the histological sections obtained from macular dystrophy, in which β-glucuronidase is lacking.

An enzymatic therapy would seem to have a future in the treatment of macular dystrophy of the cornea.

BIBLIOGRAPHY

Allison, A.C. & Dingle, J.T. Role of lysosomes in adrenal necrosis caused by dimenthyl-benzantracene. *Nature,* 209: *303-304,* (1966).

Allison, A.C. & Mallucci, L. Uptake of hydrocarbon carcinogens by lysosomes. *Nature,* 203: *1024-1027* (1964a).

Allison, A.C. & Mallucci, L. Lysosomes in dividing cells, with special reference to lymphocytes. *Lancet* ii, *1371-1375* (1964b).

Allison, A.C. & Malluci, L. Histochemical studies of lysosomes and lysosomal enzymes in virus-infected cell cultures. *J. Exptl. Med.,* 121: *463-476,* (1965a).

Allison, A.C. & Paton, G.R. Chromosomes damage in human diploid cells following activation of lysosomal enzymes. *Nature,* 207: *1170-1173,* (1965b).

Allison, A.C. & Young, M.R. Uptake of dyes and drugs by living cells in culture. *Life Sci.,* 3: *1407-1414* (1964c).

Allison, A.C. & Young, M.R. Vital staining and fluorescence microscopy of lysosomes. In: Lysosomes in Biology and Pathology. Ed. by Dingle J.T. & Fell H.B. North-Holland Publ. Comp., Amsterdam-London, pp. *600-628* (1973).

Anderson, T.F. Physical techniques in biological research. Acad. Press, New York, 1966.

Atkins, E.D.T. & Isaac, D.H. X-ray diffraction studies on the connective tissue poly-saccharides. Molecular conformations of dermatan sulphate. *J. Mol. Biol.,* 80: *773-779* (1973).

Barret, J.T. & Dingle, J.T. A lysosome component capable of binding cations and carcinogen. *Biochem. J.,* 105: 20 P. (1968).

Bastos, A.L., Terrinha, A.M., Vigario, J.D. & Mora-Nunez, J.F.U.V. induced changed in lysosomes tagged with quinacrine. *Exptl. Cell Res.,* 42: *84-88* (1966).

Basu, P.K., Miller, I. & Ormsby, H.L. Sex-chromatin as a biologic cell marker. *Amer. J. Ophthal.,* 49: *513-515* (1960).

Blum, J.D. Relations entre les dégénérescences hérédofamiliales et les opacités congéni-tales de la cornée. Etude clinique et généalogique. *Ophthalmologica,* Basel, 109, *123-136* (1945).

Blümcke, S., Thiel, H.J. & Niedorf, H.R. Licht- und Elektronenmikroskopische Unter-suchungen über die fleckförmige Hornhautdystrophie. *Ophthalmologica* (Basel), 164: *35-49* (1972).

Bucklers, M. Die erblichen Hornhautdystrophien. Klin. Mbl. Augenheilk., supp. 3: *1* (1938).

Čejková, J., Lojda, Z., Obenberger, J. & Havránková, E. Alkali burns of the rabbit cornea. I. A histochemical study of β-glucuronidase, β-galactosidase and N-acetyl-β-D-glucosaminidase. *Histochemistry,* 45: *65-69* (1975a).

Čejková, J., Lojda, Z., Obenberger, J. & Havránková, E. Alkali burns of the rabbit cornea. II. A histochemical study of glycosaminoglycans. *Histochemistry,* 45: *71-75* (1975b).

Cockeram, A.M.; Basu, P.K. and Ormsby, H.L. Viability of corneal epithelium and fibroblasts after long-term storage. *Amer. J. Ophthal.,* 43: *380-384* (1957).

Cotlier, F. & Hughes, W.F. Enzymatic deficiency in macular corneal dystrophy of the cornea (Groenouw II). Arvo Spring Meeting, Saratosa (1972).

Coulombre, A.J. The role of intraocular pressure in the development of the chick eye. II Control of corneal size. *Arch. Ophthal.* (Chicago), 57: *250-253* (1957).
Coulombre, A.J. & Coulombre, J.L. Corneal development. II. Transparency changes during rapid hydration. *Amer. J. Ophthal.*, 46: *276-280* (1958).
Coulombre, A.J. & Coulombre, J.L. The development of the structural and optical properties of the cornea. In: Smelser 'The structure of the eye', Acad. Press, N.Y.-London (1961).
Dededimos, P. On Gröenouw keratitis. *Bull. Soc. hellén ophtal.*, 17: *246* (1950).
De Duve, C. The lysosomes in retrospect. In: Lysosomes in biology and pathology. Ed. J.T. Dingle and H.B. Fell. North-Holland Publ. Comp., Amsterdam-London, 14: *3-40* (1973).
De Robertis, E., Nowinsky, V.W. & Saez, L. Cell biology. Ed. by W.B. Saunders Comp., Philadelphia (1970).
Dingle, J.T. Lysosomes. A laboratory handbook. North-Holland Publ. Comp., Amsterdam-London (1972).
Dingle, J.T. and Barret, A.J. Some special methods for the investigation of the lysosomal system. In: Lysosomes in biology and pathology. Ed. by Dingle J.T. and Fell H.B. North-Holland Publ. Comp., Amsterdam-London, pp. *555-566* (1973a).
Dingle, J.T. & Fell, H.B. Lysosomes in biology and pathology. North-Holland Publ. Comp., Amsterdam-London, American Elsevier Publ. Co., New York (1969-1973b).
Dohlman, C.H. Metabolism of the corneal graft. In: 'The transparency of cornea', (S. Duke-Elder & E.S. Perkins, eds.) Blackwell, Oxford (1960).
Draheim, J., McPherson, S.D., Evans, V.J. & Earle, W.R. Further studies on the viability of frozen corneas as determined in tissue culture. *Amer. J. Ophthal.*, 4: *182-185* (1957).
Duke-Elder, S. System of ophthalmology. Vol. II. The anatomy of the visual system. Henry Kimpton (1961).
Duke-Elder, S. System of ophthalmology. Vol. VIII, Part II (Diseases of the outer eye). Henry Kimpton, London (1961).
Dunnington, J.H. Tissue responses in ocular wounds. *Amer. J. Ophthal.*, 43: *667-678* (1957).
Dunnington, J.H. & Smelser, G.K. Incorporated S^{35} in healing wounds in normal and devitalized corneas. *Arch. Ophthal.* (Chicago), 60: *116-129* (1958).
Ehrlich, G & Halbert, S.P. The effects of anti-cornea and anti-heart serum on cultured cells of rabbit cornea and other tissues. *J. Immunol.*, 86: *267-289* (1961).
Elleder, M. Prolonged methanol fixation of soluble mucosubstances in mucopolysaccharidoses. *Histochemistry*, 46: *161-165* (1976).
Favard, P. The Golgi apparatus. In: Handbook of molecular cytology. Ed. A. Lima de Faria. North-Holland Research monographs Frontiers of Biology. North-Holland Publ. Comp., Amsterdam, 15: *1130-1155* (1969).
Fehr, Über familiäre fleckige Hornhautentartung. *Zbl. prakt. Augenheilk.*, 28: *1* (1904).
Fitton-Jackson, S. In: 'Connective Tissue'. CIDMS Symposium (R.E. Tunbridge eds.) pp. 77. Blackwell, Oxford (1957).
Fitton-Jackson, S. In: 'The cell'. Ed. by Brachet J. and Mirsky A.E., Acad. Press, London-New York, pp. *387-520* (1964).
Fowle, A.M.C. & Ormsby, H.L. Growth of cornea in tissue culture. *Amer. J. Ophthal.*, 39: *242-246* (1955).
Franceschetti, A. & Babel, J. Essai de classification anatomique des dégénérescences familiales de la cornée. *Ophthalmologica*, 109: *169-202* (1945).
Franceschetti, A. & Forni, S. The heredofamilial degenerations of the cornea: clinical aspects. Acta XVI Concilium Ophthal., vol. I: *193-244* (1950).
François, J. Heredo-familial corneal dystrophies. *Trans. Ophthal. Soc. U.K.*, 86: *367-416* (1966).
François, J. Heredofamiliäre Hornhautdystrophien. Bericht über die 71. Zusammenkunft der Deutschen Ophthalm. Gessellschaft (Heidelberg) pp. *171-222* (1971).

189

François, J. & Feher, J. Collagenolysis and regeneration in corneal burnings. *Ophthalmologica*, 165: *137-152* (1972a).

François, J. & Feher, J. Light microscopical and polarisation optical study of the macular dystrophy of the cornea. *Ophthalmologica*, 164: *19-34* (1972b).

François, J. & Feher, J. Polarisation optical investigations on the submicroscopic structure of the corneal and scleral fibrocyte cell membrane. *Ophthalmic Res.*, 4: *76-90* (1972c).

François, J., Hanssens, M. & Victoria-Troncoso, V. L'intérêt de la lumière polarisée en histologie oculaire. *Bull. Soc. Belge Ophtal.*, 144: *806-818* (1966).

François, J., Hanssens, M. & Victoria-Troncoso, V. L'intérêt de la lumière polarisée en histologie oculaire. *Ann. Oculist.* (Paris), 200: *953-976* (1967).

François, J., Hanssens, M., Tenchi, H. & Sebruijns, M. Ultrastructural findings in corneal macular dystrophy (Groenouw II type). *Opthal. Res.*, 7: *80-89* (1975a).

François, J., Hanssens, M. & Victoria-Troncoso, V. L'intérêt de la lumière polarisée en histologie oculaire. *Ann. Oculist.* (Paris), 200; *953-976* (1967).

François, J. & Rabaey, M. Recherches histo-chimiques sur le mucoïde de la cornée. *Bull. Soc. Belge Ophtal.*, 102: *1-16* (1952).

François, J., Rabaey, M. & Van der Meersche, G. L'ultrastructure de la cornée et de la sclérotique au microscope électronique. *Bull. Soc. Franç. Ophtal.*, 66: *301-315* (1953).

François, J., Rabaey, M. & Van der Meersche, G. L'ultrastructure de tissus oculaires au microscope électronique. II. Etude de la cornée et de la sclérotique. *Ophthalmologica*, 127: *74-85* (1954).

François, J. & Victoria-Troncoso, V. Transplantation of Vitreous Cell Culture. *Ophthal. Res.*, 4: *270-280* (1972d).

François, J. & Victoria-Troncoso, V. Les keratocytes activés. *Ann. Oculist.*, (Paris), 207: *811-819* (1974a).

François, J. & Victoria-Troncoso, V. Physiopathologie du kératocyte dans les dystrophies tachetée et grillagée de la cornée. Symposium sur la Cornée, XX° Congrès International d'Ophtalmologie-Paris (France) (1974b).

François, J. & Victoria-Troncoso, V. Histopathogenic study of the macular dystrophy of the cornea. *Ophthalmic Res.*, 7: *261-269* (1975b).

François, J., Victoria-Troncoso, V. & Bastos-Albarrán, E. Structure histochimique des fibres vitréennes au microscope par contraste de phase. *Bull. Soc. Belge Ophtal.*, 152: *464-471* (1969).

François, J., Victoria-Troncoso, V. & Bastos-Albarrán, E. The histochemical structure of the vitreous fibers studied by phase contrast microscopy. *Amer. J. Ophthal.*, 69: *763-773* (1970).

François, J., Victoria-Troncoso, V. & Eeckhout, M. Microscopical and histochemical study of keratocytes in culture. *Exp. Eye Res.*, 15: *471-483* (1973).

François, J., Victoria-Troncoso, V. & Zagorski, Z. Histoenzymological study of normal and pathological keratocytes in tissue culture (Macular dystrophy of the cornea). *Ophthal. Res.* 9: 357-365 (1977).

Fraser, R.D.B. & Mac Rae, T.P. Conformation in fibrous proteins and related synthetic polypeptides. Acad. Press, New York-London (1973).

Garner, A. Histochemistry of corneal macular dystrophy. *Invest. Ophthal.* 8: *475-483* (1969).

Gasic, G. & Berwick, L. Hale stain for sialic acid containing mucins. Adaptation to electron microscopy. *J. Cell. Biol.*, 19: *223-228* (1963).

Goldberg, M.F., Maumenee, A.E. & McKusick, V.A. Corneal dystrophies associated with abnormalities in the mucopolysaccharide metabolism. *Arch. Ophthal.* (Chicago), 74: *516-520* (1965).

Goldfischer, S. Demonstration of copper and acid phosphatases activity in hepatocyte lysosomes in experimental copper toxity. *Nature,*, 215: *74-75* (1967).

Goldman, G.C. & Lane, N. On the site of sulfation in the chondrocyte. *J. Cell Biol.*, 21: *353-366* (1964).

Groenouw, A. Knötchenförmige Hornhauttrübungen (noduli cornea). *Arch. Augenheilk.*, 21: *281* (1890).

190

Halbert, S.P. & Ehrlich, G. Some aspects of immunologic factors in corneal grafts. *Invest. Ophthal.*, 1: *233-243* (1962).

Hale, C.W. Histochemical demonstration of acid polysaccharides in animal tissue. *Nature* (Lond.), 157: *802* (1946).

Hamada, R., Giraud, J.P., Graf, B. & Pouliquen, Y. Etude analytique et statistique des lamelles, des kératocytes, des fibrilles de collagène de la région centrale de la cornée humaine normale (Microscopie optique et électronique). *Arch. Ophtal.* (Paris), 32: *563-570* (1972).

Hanna, C. & O'Brien, J.E. Thymidine-tritium labeling of the elements of the corneal stroma. *Arch. Ophthal.* (Chicago), 66: *362-365* (1961).

Harper, J.Y. & Pomerat, C.M. In vitro observations on the behaviour of conjunctival and corneal cells in relation to electrolytes. *Amer. J. Ophthal.*, 46: *269-276* (1958).

Harris, J.E. The physiological control of corneal hydration. *Amer. J. Ophthal.*, 44: *262-280* (1957).

Heers, H.G. & Van Hoof, F. Lysosomes and storage diseases. Acad. Press, New York-London (1973).

Hermann, J. & Meythaler, H. Licht- und elektronenmikroskopische untersuchungen bei dystrophia corneae maculosa. *Graefes Arch. Ophthal.*, 181: *165-178* (1971).

Hoffman, P. & Mashburn, T.A. Jr. Collagen-proteoglycans interaction in bovine nasal cartilage. In: Chemistry and molecular biology of the intercellular matrix. Ed. by E.A. Balazs. Acad. Press, London-New York, 2: *1179-1195* (1970).

Hoof, D. Tissue research and cell culture of the cornea. *Amer. J. Ophthal.*, 31: *709-712* (1948).

Jackus, M.A. Studies on the cornea. I. The fine structure of the rat cornea. *Amer. J. Ophthal.*, 38: *40-53* (1954).

Jackus, M.A. The fine structure of the human cornea. In: The structure of the eye. G.K. Smelser, Acad. Press, pp. *343-366* (1961).

Jackus, M.A. Further observations on the fine structure of the cornea. *Invest. Ophthal.*, 1: *202-225* (1962).

Jacobson, B. The biosynthesis of hyaluronic acid. In: Chemistry and Molecular Biology of the intercellular matrix. Ed. by E.A. Balazs, Acad. Press, London-New York, 2: *763-781* (1970).

John, I. Knotchenförmige Veränderungen der Hornhautrückfläche bei Groenouwscher familiärer Hornhautdystrophie. *Zbl. Augenheilk.*, 65: *240* (1928).

Jones, S.T. & Zimmerman, L.E. Macular dystrophy of the cornea (Groenouw type II): Clinicopathologic report of two cases with comments concerning its differential diagnosis from lattice dystrophy (Haab Dimmer). *Amer. J. Ophthal.*, 47: *1-16* (1959).

Jones, S.T. & Zimmerman, L.E. Histopathologic differentiation of granular macular and lattice dystrophies of the cornea. *Amer. J. Ophthal.*, 51: *394-410* (1961).

Kaufman, H.E., Capella, J.A. & Robbins, J.E. A study of enzyme activity in corneal repair. *Invest. Ophthal.*, 3: *34-46* (1964).

Keates, R.H. & Cvintal, T. Congenital hereditary corneal dystrophy. *Amer. J. Ophthal.*, 60: *892-894* (1965).

Kitano, S. Cytoplasmic granules of the corneal stroma cells. *Invest. Ophthal.*, 5: *277-287* (1966).

Kitano, S. Cytoplasmic granules of keratocytes and their relationships to formation of the ground substance. In: The Cornea. Macromolecular organization of a connective tissue. Ed. by M.E. Langham, The John Hopkins Press, pp. *133-143* (1969).

Kitano, S. & Goldman, J.N. Cytologic and histochemical changes in corneal wound repear. *Arch. Ophthal.* (Chicago), 76: *345-354* (1966).

Klintworth, G.K. & Vogel, F.S. Macular corneal dystrophy. An inherited acid muco-polysaccharide storage disease of the corneal fibroblast. *Amer. J. Pathol.*, 45: *565-586* (1964).

Koenig, H. The autofluorescence of the lysosomes. Its value for identification of lysosomal constituents. *J. Histochem. Cytochem.*, 11: *556-557* (1963a).

Koenig, H. Intravital staining of lysosomes by basic dyes and metabolic ions. *J. Histochem. Cytochem.*, 11: *120-121*, (1963b).

Krwawicz, T. The reticulo-endothelial system of the cornea. *Brit. J. Ophthal.*, 31: *421-423* (1947).

Lampert, I.A. & Lewis, P.D. Staining of sulphatides in metachromatic leukodystrophy with Alcian blue at high salt concentrations. *Histochemistry*, 43: *269-273* (1975).

Laurent, T.C. Structure of hyaluronic acid. In: Chemistry and Molecular Biology of the intercellular matrix. Ed. by E.A. Balazs. Acad. Press, London-New York, 3: *1421-1445* (1970).

Laurent, T.C. & Anseth, A. Studies on corneal polysaccharides. II. Characterization. *Exp. Eye Res.*, 1: *99-105* (1961).

Lev, R. & Spicer, S.S. Specific staining of sulphate groups with alcian blue at low pH. *J. Histochem. Cytochem.*, 12: *309* (1964).

Lojda, Z. Histochemical methods for acid β-galatosidase. Technics for semipermeable membranes. *Histochemie*, 37: *375-378* (1973).

Lojda, Z. Topochemistry of β-glycosidases in the aorta and coronary arteries of rats, guinea-pigs and rabbits under normal conditions and after cholesterol feeding. *Cs. Path.*, 10: *1-9* (1974).

Lorenzetti, D.W.C. & Kaufman, H.E. Macular and lattice dystrophies and their recurrence after keratoplasty. *Trans. Amer. Ophthal. and Otol.*, 71: *112-118* (1967).

Lowther, D.A., Toole, B.P. & Herrington, A.C. Interactions of proteoglycans and tropocollagen. In: Chemistry and Molecular Biology of the intercellular matrix. Ed. by E.A. Balazs, Acad. Press, London-New York, 2: *1133-1153* (1970).

Lucas, D.R. Special cytology of the eye. In: 'Cells and tissues in culture, methods, biology and physiology'. Ed. by E.N. Willmer Acad. Press, London-New York, pp. *457-520* (1965).

Malbran, E. Corneal dystrophies: a clinical, pathological and surgical aproach. *Trans. Amer. Acad. Ophthal. and Otol.*, 76: *573-624* (1972).

Malbran, E. & Victoria-Troncoso, V. Distrofias corneales, su correlación anatomoclínica, genética y quirúrgica. *An. Inst. Barraquer*, 11: *260-334* (1973).

Manual of histologic and special staining technics. Armed Forces Institute of pathology (Second edition). The Blakiston Division, McGraw-Hill Book Comp. Inc., New York-Toronto-London (1960).

Mareel, M., Dragonetti, C. & Van Peteghem, M.C. Cytochemistry of Colloidal Iron binding to the surface of Hela Cells and Human Erythrocytes. *Histochemistry* 48: *71-80* (1976).

Mathews, M.B. Molecular organization of connective tissue matrix. In: The Cornea. Macromolecular organization of a connective tissue. Ed. by M. Langham, John Hopkins Press, Baltimore, pp. *107-121* (1969).

Mathews, M.B. The interactions of proteoglycans and collagen model systems. In: Chemistry and Molecular Biology of the intercellular matrix. Ed. by E.A. Balazs, Acad. Press, London-New York, 3: *1485-1502* (1970).

Matsui, J. Über die 'in vitro' Kultur des endothels der membrana Descemetii. *Arch. Exp. Zellforsch.*, 8: *533-546* (1928-29).

Módis, L. Topo-optical investigations of mucopolysaccharides. (acid glycosaminoglycans). Polysaccharides. II. In: Handbuch der Histochemie (Graumann u. Neumann, Hrsg.) S. *11-15* Stuttgart: Gustav Fischer, Verlag (1974).

Morgan, G. Macular dystrophy of the cornea. *Brit. J. Ophthal.*, 50: *57-67* (1966).

Morrison, R.I.G. The breakdown of proteoglycans by lysosomal enzymes and its specific inhibition by an antiserum to cathepsin D. In: Chemistry and Molecular Biology in the intercellular matrix. Ed. by E.A. Balazs. Acad. Press, New York-London, 3: *1683-1706* (1970).

Mortelmans, R. & Sebruyns, M. De histologische veranderingen van de pancreas van de Cavia na intoxikatie met B.Z. 55, aangetoond door fluorochromering met Acridine-Orange. Biologisch Jaarboek, dertigste jaargang, pp. *161-170* (1962).

Movat, H.Z. Silver impregnation methods for electron microscopy. *Amer. J. Clin. Path.*, 35: *528-537* (1961).

Mowry, R.W. The special value of methods that color both acidic and vicinal hydroxyl groups in the histochemical study of mucins. With revised directions for the colloidal iron stain, the use of alcian blue G8X and their combinations with periodic acid-Schiff reaction. *Ann. N.Y. Acad. Sci.*, 106: *402-423* (1963).

Musy, J.P., Sprumont, P., Módis, L. & de Blasi, V. Ultrastructure du mucus (cellules calciformes du colon) et des granulations des mastocytes du colon. *Histochemie*, 30: *40-59* (1972).

Naylor, E.J. Polarized light studies of corneal structure. *Brit. J. Ophthal.*, 37: *77-84* (1953).

Neutra, M. & Leblond, C.P. The Golgi apparatus. *Scient. Amer.*, 220: *100-107* (1969). H3 'and glucose-H3 in the Golgi region of various cells secreting glyco-proteins or mucopolysaccharides. *J. Cell Biol.*, 30: *137-145* (1966).

Neutra, M. & Leblond, C.P. The Golgi apparatus. *Scient. Amer.*, 220: *100-107* (1969).

Obrink, B. Studies on the electrostatic interaction between collagen and chondroitin-4-sulfate. In: Chemistry and Molecular Biology in the intercellular matrix. Ed. by E.A. Balazs. Acad. Press, London-New York, 2: *1171-1178* (1970).

Offret, G. The histo-pathology of the corneal graft. In: Corneal Grafts. Ed. by B.W. Rycroft. Butterworth, London (1955).

Offret, G., Payrau, P., Pouliquen, Y., Faure, J.P. & Bisson, J. La structure fine de certaines dystrophies cornéennes. *Arch. Ophtal.* (Paris), 26: *171-181* (1966).

Payrau, P., Pouliquen, Y., Faure, J.P. & Offret, G. La transparence de la cornée. Le mécanisme de ses altérations. Masson et Cie., eds. (1967).

Pearse, A.G.E. Histochemistry. Theoretical and applied. Churchill Livingstone, Edinburgh and London (1972).

Peña Carillo, J. Histochemical aspects of the rabbit normal cornea and experimental corneal grafts. *Ophthalmologica*, 146: *260-267* (1963)

Peterson, M. & Leblond, C.P. Synthesis of complex carbohydrates in the Golgi region, as shown by radioautography after injection of labelled glucose. *J. Cell Biol.*, 21: *143-148* (1964).

Polack, F.M. Morphology of the cornea. I. Study with silver stains. *Amer. J. Ophthal.*, 51: *1051-1056* (1961).

Pratt-Johnson, J.A. Studies on the anatomy and pathology of the peripheral cornea. *Amer. J. Ophthal.*, 47: *478-488* (1959).

Prieto Diaz, H. La técnica del carbonato argéntico amoniacal de del Rio Hortega en el estudio del tejido propio de la cornea. *Arch. Histología norm. y pat.*, 3: *513-519* (1947a).

Prieto Diaz, H. La técnica del carbonato argéntico de del Rio Hortega en el estudio del tejido corneal. *Rev. med. La Plata*, 5: *23-28* (1947b).

Puchtler, H., Meloan, S.N. & Brewton, B.R. On structural formulas of basic fuchsin and aldehyde-Schiff reaction products. *Histochemistry*, 45: *255-265* (1975).

Rambourg, A., Hernandez, W. & Leblond, C.P. Detection of complex carbohydrates in the Golgi apparatus of rat cells. *J. Cell Biol.*, 40: *395-414* (1969).

Redslob, E. Traité d'ophtalmologie. Vol. I. Paris (1939).

Revel, J.P. Role of the Golgi apparatus of cartilage cells in the elaboration of matrix glycosaminoglycans. In: Chemistry and Molecular Biology of the intercellular matrix. Ed. by E.A. Balazs, Acad. Press, London-N.Y., 3: *1485-1502* (1970).

Rinehart, J.F. & Abul-Haj, S.K. An improved method for histological demonstration of acid mucopolysaccharide in tissues. *A.M.A. Arch. Pathol.*, 52: *189-194* (1951).

Robb, R.M. & Kuwabara, T. Corneal wound healing. I. The movement of polymorphonuclear leukocytes into corneal wounds. *Arch. Ophthal.* (Chicago), 68: *636-642* (1962).

Robb, R.M. & Kuwabara, T. Corneal wounds healing. II. An autoradiographic study of the cellular components. *Arch. Ophthal.* (Chicago) 72: *401-408* (1964).

Robbins, E., Marcus, P.I. & Gonatas, N.K. Dynamics of acridine orange-cell interaction II Dye induced ultrastructural changes in multivesicular bodies (acridine orange particles). *U. Cell Biol.*, 21: *49-61* (1964).

Rohem, J.N. Experimental studies on the trabecula meshwork in primates. *Arch. Ophthal.* (Chicago), 69: *335-349* (1963).

Romhanyi, G. Functional and submicroscopic structure of renal tubular epithelium. *Kisérl. Orvostud.*, 1: *73-79* (1949).

Romhányi, G. Über die submikroskopische strukturelle Grundlage der metachormatischen Reaktion. *Acta histochem.* (Jena), 15: *201-233* (1963).

Romhányi, G., Bukovinszki, A. & Déak, G. Sulfation as a collagen-specific reaction. The ultrastructure of sulfate collagen, basement membrane and reticulin fibers as shown by topo-optical reaction. *Histochemistry*, 36: *123-138* (1973).

Romhányi, G. & Bukovinszky, A. Topo-optical studies on age pigment, corpora amilacea and senile amyloid-like substance of brain. VII Internat. Congr. of Neuropathology-Budapest (1974a).

Romhányi, G & Déak, G. On the structural organization of biological membranes as shown by topooptical staining reactions. *Acta morph. Acad. Sci. hung.*, 17: *245-272* (1969).

Romhányi, G., Déak, G. & Fischer, J. Aldehyde bisulfite-toluidine blue (ABT) staining as a topo-optical reaction for demonstration of linear order to vicinal OH groups in biological structures. *Histochemistry*, 43: *333-348* (1975).

Romhányi, G. & Molnár, L. Optical polarization indicates linear arrangements of rhodopsin oligosaccharide chain in rod disc membrane of frog retina. *Nature*, 249: *486-488* (1974b).

Romhányi, G., Molnár, L. & Németh, A. Ultrastructural differences in cell membranes of erytrocytes, myeloid and lymphoid cells as shown by topo-optical reactions. *Histochemistry*, 39: *261-276* (1974c).

Rovasio, R.A., Lis, D. & Monis, B. Histochemistry and ultrastructure of the cell surfaces of the guinea pig kidney with quantitative data on carbohydrate components of glycosaminoglycans of kidney. *Histochemistry*, 40: *241-251* (1974).

Sames, K. Altersabhängige anfärbung der sauren mucopolysaccharide menschlicher rippenknorpel mit Alcianblau-acridinorange nach verschiedenen fixierungen. *Histochemistry*, 39: *277-287* (1974).

Sarkar, P., Basu, P.K. & Miller, I. Karyologic studies on cells from rabbit cornea and other tissues grown in vitro. *Invest. Ophthal.* 1: *33-40* (1962).

Saunders, A.M. Histochemical identification of acid mucopolysaccharides with acridine orange. *J. Histochem. Cytochem.*, 12: *164-170* (1964).

Scorcia, G. Moderni aspetti ultrastrutturali della membrana corneale. Acta 55 Congresso Nazionale Società Oftalmologica Italiana. 'Problemi attuali di Fisio-Patologia Corneale', pp. *17-34* (1973).

Scott, J.E. P.T.A. 'Schiff reactive' but not a glycol reagent. *J. Histochem. Cytochem.*, 21: *1084* (1973).

Scharenberg, K. The cells and nerves of the human cornea. A study with silver carbonate. *Amer. J. Ophthal.*, 40: *368-379* (1955).

Scheuner, G. & Hutschenreiter, J. Polarisationsmikroskopie in der Histophysik., S. *126-130*. Leipzig: G. Thieme (1972).

Schmidt, W.J. Der wandel der optischen anisotropie bei topochemischen reaktionen histologischer strukturen. *Ber. oberhess Ges. Natur.- u. Heilkunde, Naturwiss. Abt.*, 23: *56-85* (1947).

Seifter, S. & Gallop, P.M. The structure proteins. In: The proteins composition, structure and function. Vol. IV. pp. *153-458*. Ed. by Hans Neurath. Acad. Press, N.Y.-London (1968).

Seitz, R. & Goslar, H.G. Beitrag zur Klinik, Morphologie und Histochemie der verschiedenen formen von Hornhautdystrophie. *Klin. Mbl. Augenheilk.*, 147: *673-691* (1965).

Serafini-Fracassin, A., Wells, P. & Smith, J.W. Studies on the interaction between glycosamino-glycans and fibrillar collagen. In: Chemistry and Molecular biology of the intercellular matrix. Ed. by E.A. Balazs. Acad. Press., London-New York, 21: *1201-1215* (1970).

Smelser, G.K. Relation of factors involved in maintenance of optical properties of cornea to contact lens wear. *Arch. Ophthal.* (Chicago), 47: *328-349* (1952).

194

Smelser, G.K. & Ozanics, V. Distribution of radioactive sulfate in the developing eye. *Amer. J. Ophthal.*, 44: *102-110* (1957).
Smelser, G.K. & Ozanics, V. Morphologic and functional development of the cornea. *Amer. J. Ophthal.*, 47: *100-101* (1959).
Snip, R.C., Kenyon, K.R. & Green, W.R. Macular corneal dystrophy: ultrastructural pathology of corneal endothelium and Descemet's membrane. *Invest. Ophthal.*, 12: *88-97* (1973).
Söltz-Szöts, J. & Németz, U.R. Kritische Bemerkungen zur Gewebs-Kultur menschlicher Hornhaut. *V. Graefes Arch. Ophthal.*, 164: *86-94* (1961).
Spicer, S.S., Horn, R.G. & Leppi, T.J. Histochemistry of connective tissue mucopolysaccharides. The Connective Tissue. *pp. 251-303*. Baltimore: Williams & Wilkins Co. (Eds. Wagner, B.M. and Smith, D.E.) (1967).
Stocker, F.W., Eiring, A., Georgiade, M.S.R. & Georgiade, N. A tissue culture technique for growing corneal epithelial, stromal and endothelial tissues separetely. *Amer. J. Ophthal.*, 46: *294-298* (1958).
Stocker, F.W., Eiring, A., Georgiade, M.S.R. & Georgiade, N. Evaluation of viability of preserved rabbit corneas by tissue culture procedures. *Amer. J. Ophthal.*, 47: *772-782* (1959).
Stocker, F.W., Matton, M.T., Eiring, A., Georgiade, R. & Georgiade, N. Long-term preservation of donnor tissue for corneal grafting: correlation of results from tissue cultures with those from experimental graftings. *Amer. J. Ophthal.*, 49: *729-740* (1960).
Strauss, W. Lysosomes, phagosomes and related particles. In: 'Enzymes cytology'. Ed. by D.B. Roodijn. Acad. Press, London-New York, pp. *239-319* (1967).
Sverdlick, J. Estudio de los queratocitos con la impregnación argéntica panóptica del Rio Hortega. Acta XVII Intern. Congr. Ophthal., Montreal-New York. Vol. III pp. *1887-1892* (1954).
Swann, D.A. On the state of hyaluronic acid in a connective tissue matrix. In: Chemistry and Molecular Biology of the intercellular matrix. Ed. by E.A. Balazs. Acad. Press, London-New York, 2: *743-748* (1970).
Sykes, J.H.J. & Girard, L.J. Heterologous corneal transplants in rabbits. *Amer. J. Ophthal.*, 48: *259-262* (1959).
Takeuchi, T. & Tanoue, M. Modified lead nitrate method for acid phosphatase. In: E.A.G. Pearse's 'Histochemistry' Theoretical and applied. J. and A. Churchill Ltd. London, pp. *728-729* (1968).
Teng, C.C. Macular dystrophy of the cornea: A histochemical and electron microscopic study. *Amer. J. Ophthal.*, 62: *436-454* (1966).
Thiel, H.J., Henke, H. & Caesar, R. Klinik und Pathologie der fleckförmigen Hornhautdystrophie. *Klin. Mbl. Augenheilk.*, 150: *387-390* (1971).
Thines-Sempoux, D. Chemical similarities between the lysosomes and plasma membranes. *Biochem. J.*, 105: *20-21* (1968).
Thines-Sempoux, D. A comparison between the lysosomal and the plasma membrane. In: Lysosomes in biology and pathology. Ed. by Dingle J.T. and Fell H.B., North-Holland Pub. Comp., London-Amsterdam, vol. 3: pp. *287-299* (1973).
Threadgold, L.T. The ultrastructure of the animal cell. Pergamon Press, Oxford (1969).
Thygeson, P. Cultivation in vitro of human conjunctival and corneal epithelium. *Amer. J. Ophthal.*, 22: *649-654* (1939).
Van Canneyt, J. & Kluyskens, J. Dystrophie cornéenne heredofamiliale (Type Groenouw). *Bull. Soc. Belge Ophtal.*, 89: *351-355*, (1948).
Varga, M. & Feher, J. Polarizing microscopic studies on the regeneration behaviour of perforating corneal wounds. *Acta Ophthal. Kbh.*, 48: *1080-1090* (1970).
Victoria-Troncoso, V. & Malbran, E. Recherche histochimique sur la dystrophie oedémateuse congénitale de la cornée (rapport avec les mucopolysaccharidoses). *Bull. Soc. Belge Ophtal.*, 151: *411-426* (1969).
Vidal, B.C. de, & Mello, S. Macromolecular conformation of the colon mucus as re-

vealed by detection of anisotropic phenomena. *Ann. Histochem.*, 19: *151-156* (1974).

Virchow, H. Mikroskopische Anatomie de aüsseren Augenhaut und des Lidaparates. Graefes-Saemich Handbuch der Gesamten Augenheilkunde, Eingelmann, Leipzig (1910).

Wattiaux, R. Biochemistry and function of lysosomes. In: Lima de Faria A., 'Handbook of molecular cytology', North-Holland Pub. Comp., Amsterdam, pp. *1159-1178* (1969).

Weimar, V.L. The sources of fibroblasts in corneal wounds repair. A quantitative analysis. *Arch. Ophthal.* (Chicago), 60: *93-109* (1958).

Weimar, V.L. Activation of corneal stromal cells to take up the vital dye neutral red. *Exp. Cell Res.*, 18: *1-14* (1959).

Weimar, V.L. Effect of animo acid, purine and pyrimidine analogues on activation of corneal stromal cells to take up neutral red. *Invest. Ophthal.*, 1: *226-232* (1962).

Weimar, V.L. & Haraguchi, K.H. The development of enzyme activities in corneal connective tissue cells during the lag phase of wound repair. I. 5-nucleotidase and succinic dehydrogenase. *Invest. Ophthal.*, 4: *853-866* (1965).

Weimar, V.L. & Haraguchi, K.H. The development of enzyme activities in corneal connective tissue cells during the lag phase of wound repair. II. Formalin-resistant oxidase-like reaction. *Invest. Ophthal.*, 5: *14-21* (1966).

Wolter, R.J. Innervation of the corneal endothelium of the eye of the rabbit. *Arch. Ophthal.* (Chicago), 58: *246-250* (1957).

Wolter, R.J. Reactions of the cellular elements of the corneal stroma. *Arch. Ophthal.*, (Chicago), 59: *873-881* (1958).

Wolter, R.J. The trabecular endothelium. Its degeneration in closure of the chamber angle. *Arch. Ophthal.* (Chicago), 61: *928-938* (1959).

Yamada, K. The chemical cytology of the mouse parathyroid gland. *Z. Zellforsch.*, 65: *805-831* (1965).

Yamada, K. & Ukai, M. The histochemistry of mucosaccharides in some organs of germfree rats. *Histochemistry*, 47: *219-238* (1976).

Yamada, K. & Yokote, M. Morphochemical analysis of mucosubstances in some epithelial tissues of the cel (Anguilla japonica). *Histochemistry*, 43: *161-172* (1975).

Zelenin, A.V. Fluorescence microscopy of lysosomes and related structures in living cells. *Nature*, 212: *425-426* (1966).

SUBJECT INDEX